ESCAPE THE DIET TRAP

Emily —

Have really enjoyed
reading your blog
(thanks for writing it!)

Hope you like the book!

Kind regards

John.

DR JOHN BRIFFA

ESCAPE THE DIET TRAP

Lose weight for good without
calorie-counting, extensive
exercise or hunger

FOURTH ESTATE • *London*

First published in Great Britain in 2012 by
Fourth Estate
An imprint of HarperCollins*Publishers*
77–85 Fulham Palace Road
London W6 8JB

Typeset in Sabon and Gill Sans by G&M Designs Limited,
Raunds, Northamptonshire
Printed and bound in Great Britain by
Clays Ltd, St Ives plc

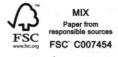

MIX
Paper from
responsible sources
FSC
www.fsc.org   FSC™ C007454

CONTENTS

ESCAPE THE DIET TRAP: AN OVERVIEW

Many of us will know what it's like to fight a losing battle with our weight, and rates of obesity are ballooning. Yet we're assured that the solution to our plus-sized problem is simple: all we need to do is 'eat less and exercise more'. This advice seems to make sense. The trouble is, not only our collective experience but scientific research, too, shows that applying this advice hardly ever brings significant weight loss in the long term.

The usual explanation offered here is that those who fail with conventional tactics lack willpower and self-control. The reality, though, is that calorie-based strategies for slimming not only don't work, but simply *can't* work, for all but a small minority.

Escape the Diet Trap explores the reasons why traditional approaches to weight loss are a crashing failure. It reveals how eating less and exercising more causes the body to resist weight loss, and can actually predispose to weight *gain* over time. Moreover, the book offers a science-based, tried and tested approach for satisfying and sustainable weight loss that works *with* the body's physiological processes, not against them.

Applying the advice here promises permanent weight loss and enhanced health. What is more, the book shows precisely how all this can be achieved without calorie counting, portion control,

I

extensive exercise or hunger. *Escape the Diet Trap* offers the science and real-world strategies that make healthy, sustained weight loss *easy and enjoyable*.

1. Diets Don't Work

We know that diets don't work, and this chapter reviews the results of studies of conventional dieting, with or without exercise, over time. Research reveals that, even in the very overweight, eating less and exercising more bring average losses of no more than a few pounds in the long term.

2. The Obesity Paradox

The body mass index (BMI) is the most commonly used measure of weight, and we're urged to conform to normal and 'healthy' BMI levels. This chapter reveals why the BMI, although popular, is a wholly inadequate tool for assessing body weight. It also presents evidence that 'bigger is better' for overall health, especially as we age.

3. Toxic Waist

Recent research shows that the *location* of accumulated fat determines its likely impact on health: fat packed in and around the abdomen turns out to be the most harmful for both the body and brain. This chapter explores the risks of 'abdominal obesity', and provides guidance on how to assess and monitor this quite simply.

4. The Burning Issue

'Eating less' is a central tenet of conventional weight-loss advice. This chapter shows, though, how, when we consciously cut back on calories, the body puts a brake on its metabolism. This makes it progressively more difficult to lose weight, and can cause weight to return alarmingly quickly once food restriction is relaxed.

5. The Hunger Within

A major reason why traditional diets fail is the hunger they almost inevitably induce. In this chapter, we explore the sometimes devastating impact dieting and hunger have on psychological and general wellbeing.

6. Low-Fat Fallacy

Fat contains twice as many calories as carbohydrate or protein, and low-calorie diets therefore tend to be low in fat. Yet, as this chapter reveals, dietary fat does not drive obesity, and eating less of it is ineffective for shifting body fat. These observations are explained through an understanding of how fat stores are regulated in the body. Insights here suggest that conventional low-fat diets are possibly the worst kinds of diets if lasting weight loss is our goal.

7. Is a Calorie a Calorie?

Many weight-loss experts claim that 'a calorie is a calorie'. The idea here is that, where body weight is concerned, it's only the *number* of calories we consume not the *form* they come in that counts. Others claim, however, that some diets bring weight loss that cannot be explained by calorie content alone – the so-called 'metabolic advantage'. This chapter presents evidence for this, and reveals the sort of diet that appears to offer it.

8. Hunger No More

While some see hunger as a prerequisite for weight loss, the reality is that the *less* hungry people are, the *more* weight they tend to lose: keeping the appetite under control is what makes healthy eating easy and sustainable. In this chapter, we explore the type of diet that is most effective for keeping hunger at bay.

9. Inflammatory Arguments

Fat stores in the body are ultimately determined by the action of specific hormones. In this chapter we explore how low-level *inflammation* can disrupt hormonal functioning, and in turn may lead to weight gain. The chapter focuses on the impact of inflammation on two key hormones – insulin and leptin – and goes on to explore the role of diet in improving hormonal function and bringing about lasting weight loss.

10. Diets on Trial

Low-fat diets are the mainstay of conventional approaches to weight loss, though 'low-carb' diets have gained in popularity in recent years. There is considerable debate about which of these diets is best for weight loss. This chapter reviews a decade's worth of research into the relative effectiveness of 'low-fat' and 'low-carb' diets, and reveals the latter to be the clear winner.

11. The Primal Principle

Research reveals that low-carbohydrate diets are the best for weight loss, but what about *health?* This chapter argues that the healthiest diet for us, in theory at least, is a diet that reflects that of our hunter-gatherer ancestors. Here, we explore the diet that sustained us for the vast majority of our time on this planet, as well as the dietary detours we have taken in relatively recent times.

12. A Matter of Fat

Primally inspired nutrition tells us that saturated fat is something we should be well adapted to, yet we're warned that eating it gums up our arteries and hastens our demise. This chapter starts with a thorough analysis of the science on saturated fat and heart disease, and reveals the absence of incriminating evidence here. The chapter also explores the health effects of the other major dietary fats including monounsaturated fat and polyunsaturated fat, as well as industrially produced fats found in processed foods such as margarine.

13. The Question of Cholesterol

Cholesterol is famous for its vessel-clogging effects, and we're urged to keep levels of it under control. This chapter reviews the relationship between cholesterol and health, and reveals that our fears here are largely unfounded.

14. Grain of Truth

Grain-based foods such as bread, rice, pasta and breakfast cereals are recommended as staples in our diet, particularly in their 'whole' and unrefined forms. Yet grains are relatively recent additions to the human diet, so are they really the staff of life? In this chapter we explore the potential for starchy carbohydrates to impact on the body's chemistry in a way that actually contributes to the burden of obesity and associated ills. We also revisit the idea that eschewing grains risks us falling short in essential nutrients.

15. Sweet and Sour

This chapter explores the effects of refined sugar, including fructose and 'high fructose corn syrup', on weight and health. The chapter also investigates the supposed benefits of artificial sweeteners as an aid to weight control, and reveals research which suggests that they might actually promote weight gain over time.

16. Sacred Cow

Dairy products are widely recommended on the basis that they are essential for building healthy bones. As this chapter shows, though, neither calcium nor dairy products have much bearing on bone health. The suitability of different dairy products regarding weight control and other aspects of health is also discussed.

5

17. Appetite for Change

Following on from Chapter 8, here we explore other dietary strategies for sating the appetite, allowing us to eat *less*, without feeling hungry. The chapter focuses on the importance of blood sugar control here, as well as the avoidance of food ingredients that stimulate the appetite. A section on emotional eating is also included, as well as advice on overcoming it.

18. Prime Fuel

In this chapter, all the major foods are rated according to their effects on body weight and health. Practical recommendations regarding their consumption are made.

19. Fluid Thinking

Here, the most common beverages, including water, fruit juice, soft drinks, tea, coffee and alcohol, are assessed from a body weight and health perspective.

20. Make a Meal of It

Knowing what to eat and drink is one thing; putting our knowledge into practice can be another. This chapter offers suggestions and practical advice about healthy eating, including meal plans and snack ideas.

21. Affirmative Action

The research shows that 'aerobic' exercise such as walking, running and cycling is not effective for weight loss, and this chapter explains why. The chapter goes on to explore the benefits exercise *does* offer, and provides practical information and advice about sustainable forms of activity.

22. Going Lower

For a few, fat loss can be slow going, or they may find themselves 'plateauing' at a weight that is higher than they would like. Should slow or stalled weight loss be an issue, this chapter provides two powerful strategies for overcoming this in the form of 'intermittent fasting' and 'high-intensity intermittent exercise'.

23. Long Gone

Sticking to new-found habits can be challenging sometimes, and obstacles can come up along the way. This chapter explores the common pitfalls in making and sustaining healthy changes, and how to address them using simple psychological and behavioural strategies.

24. *Escape the Diet Trap* in a Nutshell

The key insights and recommendations of the book in a handy dos and don'ts form.

25. Real-Life Stories

First-hand accounts from those who have positively transformed their weight and wellbeing easily and enjoyably.

REAL-LIFE STORIES

I'd always been a chubby chap, even when I was a kid. For most of my adult life it was just a bit of flab around my waist, so I got away with it. Like many blokes, that bit of flab started to expand when I hit my thirties, and despite various attempts to shift it with loads of exercise, calorie counting and various fad diets, at best I wouldn't get any fatter. I resigned myself to being fat.

When I hit 16 stone at the age of 37, my dad – a Type 2 diabetic – had a quiet word expressing his concern that I was going the same way as him. My dad is a man of few words, so when he talks, you listen. Suddenly, I had the motivation to do something about my ballooning weight.

I started a calorie-controlled diet one New Year. I set myself a goal of losing a pound each week until Easter, which didn't seem like too much of a stretch. But after two days, I was hungry and miserable. I couldn't see how I was doing to live like this for months. In my desperation I searched online for diet tips for men, and came across Dr John Briffa's work. Four months later I had lost 2½ stone in weight and I've maintained this new weight ever since. Most of the weight has come from my middle – my waist size has dropped from 40 to 34 inches. This has come at a price: I have had to buy an entire new wardrobe as nothing fits!

I regularly notice friends' and colleagues' jaws drop when they see me, as they genuinely cannot believe how much thinner and younger I look. I think the best things about losing weight following Dr Briffa's advice was being able to do without intensive exercise, calorie counting, or being hungry all the time.

For me, this is not a transitory diet – it's a change in lifestyle and beliefs. And it works – I haven't just lost weight, but sleep better, have more energy and feel healthier.

Mauro

For years I rubbed along at a fairly steady weight until about 18 years ago when I inexplicably started gaining weight which I found impossible to shift. I was diagnosed with an underactive thyroid, and naively thought that once the medication kicked in my metabolism would return to normal and all the extra weight would disappear. After a while, I realized this was never going to happen.

I tried every diet I could lay my hands on – cabbage soup, F-plan, South Beach, low-fat – but each one was more disappointing than the last. I was always hungry, which made me cranky, and the recommended foods were often expensive and horrid. The weight loss, if there was any, was minimal and short-term. With every failure my self-esteem plunged to even further depths. I sort of gave up

I came across Dr Briffa's work and his ideas on diet and weight loss. It was a light-bulb moment and finally, I've been able to lose weight, and specifically from where I needed to – around my middle.

I don't use scales, but know how effective this way of eating has been by the way I look and how my clothes fit. A case in point: about nine years ago I bought my 'perfect dress' on a trip to the US. It was way too small and I vowed that one day it would fit. It does now!

Roz Hubley

9

INTRODUCTION

Have you ever gone on a diet and lost weight, only subsequently to put it all back on again? Have your attempts to lose weight ever involved restricted eating or extensive exercise regimes that were simply unsustainable in the long term? Do you feel trapped in repeating cycles of weight loss and weight gain? If you've answered 'yes' to one or more of these questions, you are not alone: according to research, only a lucky few seem to be able to lose weight *and* keep it off. Shedding and regaining weight is, apparently, a national pastime.

What if I were to tell you that the conventional approach to weight loss – to 'eat less and exercise more' – is not only ineffective, but actually stands to make matters worse? How would you feel knowing that calorie-based weight-loss advice, as dispensed by our governments and health experts for decades, causes changes in the body that likely doom us to a life of excess weight and its related problems? Would you be interested to learn that there exists a science-based, tried and tested approach to *sustained* weight loss and enhanced health, that requires nothing in the way of calorie counting, extensive exercise or hunger?

These claims may sound bold to you, given what we've been assured about the cause of excess weight and how to remedy it:

11

we get fat because we consume more calories than we burn, and the solution is simply to redress the balance by cutting back on the amount we eat and upping our exercise. Yet in my work as a doctor over two decades I have met countless determined and disciplined individuals who just can't seem to crack their weight issue by 'doing the right thing'. As you'll learn in this book, it's not just this collective experience, but scientific research, too, that demonstrate how ineffective calorie-based strategies are for weight loss in the long term.

The blame for faltering fat loss is usually laid at the feet of would-be slimmers, who are assumed to be lacking the required willpower and self-control. Such judgements can be self-applied, too, of course, with many individuals berating *themselves* for 'lacking what it takes' to control their weight.

But, seeing as conventional strategies fail so miserably for practically *everyone* who tries them, it seems only right to wonder whether there's something wrong with the strategies themselves. Isn't it about time we asked some serious questions of the 'calorie principle' and the science that underpins it?

Escape the Diet Trap is part polemic, in that it challenges possibly the most widely believed health 'fact' of all: that our weight is ultimately determined by the balance of calories going into and coming out of our bodies. The book reveals how body weight is determined by much more than the mere balance of 'calories in and calories out'. Moreover, we'll see how calorie-based approaches cause the body to 'defend' its weight and hang onto fat through a variety of mechanisms. Not only can this make weight loss heavy going, it predisposes to gradually increasing weight over time. Sound familiar? While the calorie principle may have formed the basis of weight-loss advice for several decades, science shows it to be an ultimately destructive concept.

Escape the Diet Trap is practical, too: once we're clear about where the pitfalls lie, I'll reveal to you precisely how to avoid them. In these pages you will learn what science and my clinical experience with real people reveal about how to achieve successful, sustainable weight loss without consciously cutting back on food and without the need for exhausting exercise. The approaches advocated here are designed to avoid all the hazards of conventional slimming by working *with* the body's self-regulatory mechanisms, rather than *against* them.

The early part of the book examines what happens when the body is subjected to a traditional weight-reducing 'diet'. You will learn, for instance, how, when food is restricted, the body compensates by down-regulating the metabolism. This can make weight loss painfully slow, and also lead to a frustrating plateauing of weight.

Many imagine that any slowing of their metabolism can be countered by increasing their exercise efforts. *Escape the Diet Trap* reveals, though, that 'aerobic' exercises such as running, brisk walking and cycling are actually quite *in*effective for weight loss, and precisely why this is so.

The disappointment of the meagre returns that come from eating less and exercising more is made even harder to bear by the almost inevitable hunger that comes with this approach. Moreover, we'll see how even quite moderate caloric restriction can lead to an amplification in appetite that can sap the resolve and have adverse effects on our physical and mental wellbeing (you probably know the feeling).

And as if these effects were not destructive enough, you'll learn how conventional dieting puts an emphasis on foods that actually *encourage* deposition of fat in the body via well-established biochemical pathways.

It's not so much that conventional diets don't work – but more that they *can't* work.

One thing that will become clear as you read this book is that the diet so often advocated for weight loss – one restricted in calories and fat – simply does not deliver on its promise. Not only that, but you'll see how this supposedly healthy diet can actually increase your risk of conditions such as heart disease and Type 2 diabetes.

Much of the science that supports these sometimes shocking truths dates back several decades, and the obvious question therefore is why erroneous information has persisted for so long. There's no doubt that some of the misinformation is unwitting

– coming from well-meaning individuals who nonetheless remain unaware of the relevant scientific evidence in the area. I know this, because at one time I myself believed *all* of the myths I expose in this book. The problem was that my beliefs were based on what I'd been taught and heard, and accepted in good faith. Regular reviewing of the scientific literature over the last 20 years has revealed to me just how misguided and dangerous the vast majority of conventional nutritional 'wisdom' is.

Intellectual naivety may be partly to blame for the faulty nutritional notions that abound, but it's also certainly not the whole explanation. There's some truth, I think, in the idea that much misinformation is disseminated and popularized by individuals, businesses and organizations that stand to gain from it. For example, the idea that it's an excess of dietary fat that is fattening allows food companies to sell us a dizzying array of 'low-fat' or 'fat-reduced' foods that promise weight loss and health benefits. These foods, based on sugar and grain, are generally cheap to produce and offer considerable potential for profit.

If these products fail to have the desired effect (or actually contribute to the problem), then so much the better, as this just helps keep us coming back for more. Strategies that bring only transient success can help ensure our periodic attendance at weight-loss clinics or slimming clubs, too. The fact is, peddling weight-loss 'solutions' that are ultimately destined to fail is good for *business*.

Putting profit ahead of public health also explains the origin and perpetuation of many nutritional concepts that simply don't stand up to scientific scrutiny. Examples include the idea that margarine is better for us than butter, and that artificial sweeteners have benefits over sugar for weight control. Popularizing these beliefs may be good for the bottom line but, as you'll see, there really isn't a scrap of evidence to support them. Moreover, evidence exists which points to such novel foodstuffs as being damaging to health.

At the risk of sounding like an angry middle-aged man, the more dietary misinformation I've become aware of over the years, the more outraged I've found myself getting. I've seen at first hand the suffering and misery conventional nutritional advice can cause, in the form of health issues such as persistent fatigue, mood swings or depression, eating disorders, digestive disease, out-of-control diabetes and, of course, weight problems. I believe I have a responsibility to do what I can to right these wrongs, though I am not alone in this quest. Within the book, as well as in the resources section, I suggest sources of information that I believe offer trustworthy information and advice regarding diet and other health-related matters.

No amount of information means anything without action, though, and one hugely important step you can take in the right direction is to vote with your feet by eschewing suspect processed foods. This is not just a political gesture: experience tells me that putting emphasis on natural, unprocessed foods is an immensely effective tool for bringing about effortless weight loss and enhanced health.

This approach is also consistent with what common sense tells us about healthy eating: there's a strong argument for basing our diet on the foods our species has been eating longest in terms of our time on this planet. Meat, fish, eggs, nuts, fruits and vegetables are the foods we evolved to eat, after all, and are therefore those that we're best adapted to and serve our needs the best. This is not just a theory – as you'll see, there is abundant scientific evidence to support it.

For instance, the research shows quite clearly that the most effective diet for weight control is one that is richer in protein and fat and lower in carbohydrate than is traditionally advised. It's probably no coincidence that this broad dietary make-up emulates that of our evolutionary diet.

Such diets, specifically relatively high in fat and low in carbohydrate, are viewed by some as inherently unhealthy, and the expression 'fad diet' is often used to describe them. But can a diet that reflects the one that sustained us for the vast majority of our time on this planet really be described as a *fad*? Does it really make sense that the foods that nourished us for over two million years pose perilous threats to our health?

Trust me when I tell you this book is as much about health as it is about weight loss. I'm not in the business of advocating foods that might lighten your load but at the same time lessen your lifespan. *Escape the Diet Trap* goes beyond the impact diet has on weight by unpicking its relationship with health, too. The book refers to hundreds of scientific studies that demonstrate the recommendations it contains are designed not just for sustained weight loss, but enhanced health and wellbeing, too.

While the science that underpins the strategies in *Escape the Diet Trap* is extensive, I've inevitably had to be somewhat selective about what I included in the book. Some may say that such selectivity risks bias. I hold my hands up to this. Here's why …

For the vast majority of my time as a doctor I have been primarily interested in using nutrition as a way of enhancing health and reversing illness. The reason that I feel confident and enthusiastic about recommending the strategies and solutions in this book is because I have witnessed them work in practice with countless individuals.

I have seen individuals who for years have struggled with their weight finally achieve lasting, satisfying success with *ease* using the principles outlined in this book. I've known individuals liberate themselves from repeating cycles of semi-starvation and soul-destroying weight regain. I've been repeatedly struck by the joy and delight of people who have lost substantial amounts of weight without hunger or extensive exercise, restoring their health and self-esteem at the same time. Many of these individuals report that their doctors are astounded at the improvement in their weight and markers of health such as blood pressure and blood fat levels.

I readily admit that seeing countless individuals break free from 'the diet trap' and transform their health and happiness using the approaches detailed in this book has left me somewhat biased.

I wouldn't have written this book if I were not keen that people get benefit from it. My experience with legions of people over many years tells me that, by applying the advice this book offers, you stand to see a seriously positive shift in your weight, wellbeing and health. What is more, these approaches require nothing in the way of portion control, hunger or long hours spent in the gym or pounding the pavement. In short, you'll discover that lasting, health-enhancing weight loss can be *easy* – when you know how.

HOW TO USE THIS BOOK

If you read this book from cover to cover, you'll realize that the earlier chapters provide the background, much of it scientific, for the more specific and practical advice that comes later. *Escape the Diet Trap* is written in this way because understanding *why* and *how* specific approaches bring benefit helps us make and maintain positive changes in our lives.

This book undoubtedly contains much more 'science' and demands more from you than traditional weight-loss books. However, I guarantee you that the efforts you expend here will be richly rewarded in the form of a knowledge that is both deep and complete. Absorbing the key principles contained in this book will almost certainly allow you to take control of your weight for the rest of your life.

However, you may be keen to get on with things. Or perhaps you're simply not that interested in the science and research that underpins the recommendations in the book. In either case, you may want to skip a lot of theory and go to the parts of the book that are geared more to *what* to do (rather than why you might do it). In which case, I recommend you start at Chapter 18 (Prime Fuel) and read through to the end of the book.

However, if you do take this approach, I suggest you at least read the summaries at the end of each of the earlier chapters under the heading 'The Bottom Line'. Absorbing the key learning points here will, even without the detail, set the scene for the more practical information and advice later on.

Dr John Briffa
London, July 2011

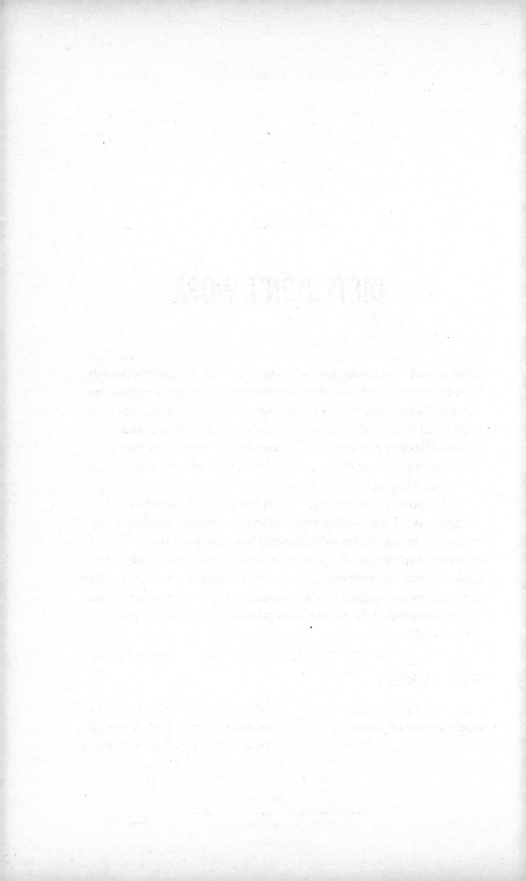

Chapter 1

DIETS DON'T WORK

Ideas about what causes obesity vary. But you'll almost certainly be familiar with the idea that, at the end of the day, the problem is a product of caloric imbalance: specifically, the consumption of calories in excess of those burned through metabolism and activity. No doubt you'll also be familiar with the idea that the solution to your weight problem is simply to redress the balance by eating less and exercising more.

The 'calorie principle' that forms the basis of conventional weight-loss advice is utterly persuasive at first glance. But a mountain of anecdotal evidence and perhaps your own experience questions its validity. In this chapter, we're going to look at what research reveals about the effectiveness of orthodox approaches to weight loss. How much weight do people lose on calorie-controlled diets, and does adding exercise make much difference?

Slim Pickings

Here we're going to use published scientific research to judge the effectiveness of conventional, calorie-based approaches to weight loss. I'm going to focus on studies that fulfil the following criteria:

1. The dietary strategies used were based on conventional approaches to weight loss, i.e. reduced calorie intake, generally with an emphasis on low-fat foods.

2. Within the study, some individuals changed only their diet, while others added exercise, too.

3. The 'intervention' (dietary restriction with or without exercise) lasted at least a year.

4. Individuals were assessed at least two years after the start of the intervention.

Limiting the studies to those where individuals were monitored for at least two years after the start of their efforts to lose weight allows us to assess the *long-term* success of these approaches. Many of us will know what it is to get a short-term win from eating less and exercising more, but it's the long game we're interested in here.

I'm going to go through each study in turn. For each, I provide a brief description of the study and its results. The study descriptions refer, among other things, to the average 'body mass index' (BMI) of the participants. This is calculated by dividing an individual's weight in kilograms by the square of their height in metres (kg/m^2). Traditionally, BMIs of 25.0 and above are regarded as 'overweight', while those of 30.0 and above are deemed 'obese'.

Study 1[1]

Individuals with an average age of 36 and average BMI of 35.0 were prescribed a calorie-reduced diet (individuals ate about 1,000 calories less each day than the amount needed to maintain a stable weight). Some of the individuals added exercise to this dietary restriction in the form of brisk walking for 45 minutes, 4–5 times each week. The intervention lasted for a year, and weight was assessed another year after the end of the intervention.

ESCAPE THE DIET TRAP

Average result:

Diet only: gain of 0.9 kg
Diet and exercise: loss of 2.2 kg

Study 2[2]

Individuals with an average age of 42 and average BMI of 36.5 were prescribed a diet offering 1,200–1,500 calories a day. Exercise, for those who added this, came in the form of regular aerobic exercise, resistance exercise (exercise designed to strengthen muscles), or some of both types of exercise. The intervention lasted 12 months, and the individuals were assessed 13 months after the end of the intervention.

Average result:

Diet only: loss of 4.6 kg
Diet and exercise: loss of 5.2 kg

Study 3[3]

Individuals with an average age of 45 and an average BMI of 36.0 were prescribed a low-fat diet containing initially 800–1,000 calories per day, rising to 1,200–1,500 calories a day for most of the two-year intervention. For those who added exercise, too, this came in the form of brisk walking for 3 miles, 5 times a week. The intervention lasted 24 months.

Average result:

Diet only: loss of 2.1 kg
Diet and exercise: loss of 2.5 kg

DIETS DON'T WORK

Study 4[4]

Individuals with an average age of 43 and average BMI of 25.5 ate a low-fat, high-carbohydrate diet for 12 months. Some of the group added exercise to this, in the form of 30 minutes or more of aerobic exercise, 4–5 times per week. Individuals were assessed a further 12 months after the end of the intervention period.

Average result:

Diet only: no change in weight
Diet and exercise: loss of 1.9 kg

STUDY	INTERVENTION LENGTH (MONTHS)	FOLLOW-UP (MONTHS)	WEIGHT CHANGE FROM DIET ONLY (KG)	WEIGHT CHANGE FROM DIET AND EXERCISE (KG)
1	12	12	-0.9	-2.2
2	12	13	-4.6	-5.2
3	24	24	-2.1	-2.5
4	12	12	0.0	-1.9
average			-1.9	-2.95

Table 1: Summary of weight losses for diet-only and diet plus exercise interventions

Two years after embarking on a long-term (lasting at least a year) restrictive dietary regime, average weight loss was in the order of just 2 kg. Even when regular exercise is added, the weight loss still only averaged about 3 kg (about 6½ lbs). These outcomes look even more paltry when put in the context of the weight of many of the study participants. For someone of average height, a BMI of 35 works out at about 16 stone. I'd say it's unlikely that individuals of this weight would view a loss of a few pounds as a satisfying return on investment in terms of their diet and exercise efforts.

While the studies examined here varied in precise design, one thing they had in common is that the participants generally had a lot of educational input and support, either individually or as part of a group. In this sense, these studies represent quite *intensive* interventions. This is in stark contrast to most individuals seeking to lose weight, who are quite often plugging away on their own. The likelihood, therefore, is that the results seen in these studies were significantly better than those achieved by people in the real world.

One thing that is clear from the evidence is that the average weight losses fell significantly short of that predicted by application of the calorie principle. I'll be explaining how this can be in subsequent chapters, particularly Chapters 4 (The Burning Issue) and 6 (Low-Fat Fallacy).

Another potential surprise is just how ineffective exercise was for the purposes of weight loss when employed as an adjunct to dietary restraint. The results from these studies suggest an additional loss of a mere 1 kg in those who were exercising regularly. Other evidence points to similarly disappointing results in this regard. For example, one review that included all the above studies as well as those of shorter duration found the same thing,[5] as did another major review of the relevant literature.[6] In Chapter 21 (Affirmative Action), I'll offer explanations for why exercise, so often advised, does little to lighten our load.

The Blame Game

It seems it really is true that diets don't work. But *why*?

Many of us have so much faith in the calorie principle that the knee-jerk response is to look for fault in those who apply it. The overwhelming belief, and one often held by health professionals, is that failed slimmers delude themselves about the eating and exercise habits or simply do not stick to the rules. Such accusations may legitimately be levelled at some, I suppose. But could the poor results be not because people don't work hard enough at 'eating less and exercising more', but because this strategy itself just doesn't work?

In subsequent chapters, I'll be exploring why applying the calorie principle actually condemns the vast majority of us to weight-loss failure in the long term. Before that, though, let's look at how body weight is conventionally assessed, and whether conforming to weight-based norms is the best thing for us.

The Bottom Line

- Dietary restriction leads to long-term weight loss in the order of 2 kg.

- Adding exercise to dietary restraint appears to improve weight loss by only about one additional kilogram.

- The consistent failure of a calorie-based approach to weight loss suggests that it is inherently ineffective.

Chapter 2

THE OBESITY PARADOX

If you have a decent amount of weight to lose, there's a good chance your doctor has warned you about the risks of excess weight and urged you to slim down. Governments and the medical profession frequently warn that being overweight or obese puts us in mortal danger, and encourage us to conform to weight norms defined by a measure known as the body mass index (BMI).

In this chapter we'll explore why the BMI, although popular, is a really quite inadequate tool for assessing individual health. We'll also examine evidence that suggests that somewhat higher BMIs than are traditionally advised may signal better overall health, particularly in later life.

Why Weight?

The BMI is the measure most commonly used by health practitioners to assess weight and its impact on health. While the BMI usually forms the basis of the advice health professionals give to individuals about their weight, there is good reason to be mistrustful of it.

The fundamental issue is that the BMI tells us nothing about body *composition*. Someone with an 'obese' BMI may indeed be

THE OBESITY PARADOX

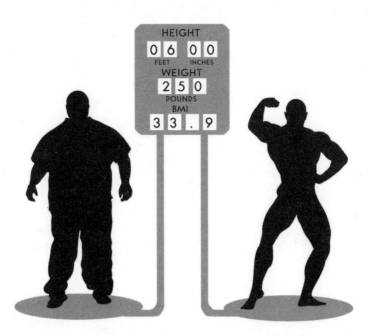

HEIGHT

0	6	0	0

FEET   INCHES

WEIGHT

2	5	0

POUNDS

BMI

3	3	.	9

Figure 1: Illustration of how body composition is not reflected in the BMI

overly fat and unhealthy. At the same time, though, it is entirely possible for someone to be in great physical shape, and solidly built from a muscle perspective, and to also have a BMI that marks them out as 'obese'. Figure 1 illustrates this point graphically. When judged according to the BMI, the two people depicted here are equally healthy. *Really?*

Does the BMI Shape Up?

It's clear that the BMI has significant limitations as a marker or guide to *individual* health, but how does it perform when applied to *groups* of people? By rights, individuals with BMIs around the middle of the 'normal' or 'healthy' range should be the healthiest.

When considering the relationship between BMI and health, it pays to take as wide a view as possible. The way to do this is to assess its relationship, not with the risk of individual conditions, but with *overall risk of death*. Ultimately, risk of death is 100 per cent, of course. In studies 'risk of death' (sometimes termed 'overall mortality' or just 'mortality') refers to likelihood of death over a specified period of time (usually many years).

The broad relationship between BMI and mortality is shown in Figure 2 below. You'll see that risk of death is higher with BMIs at both the lower and higher end of the spectrum.

The question is, does the lowest point in the curve – where risk of death is lowest – correspond to what health professionals tell us is the best BMI for us? And is being 'overweight' linked with hazards for overall health, as we're told?

In one major study, a BMI of 25.0–27.5 (technically 'overweight') was *not* associated with an increased risk of death[1] compared to BMIs in the 'healthy band'. In other research,[2] significantly enhanced risk of death was not seen until BMI values exceeded 30.0. Further questions regarding the wisdom of the traditional BMI bands are asked by the results of studies which show a link between 'overweight' BMIs and actually *reduced* risk of death.[3,4]

One thing that has come out of the research is that the relationship between BMI and mortality is influenced to some degree by age. In one study,[5] being 'overweight' was associated with an enhanced risk of death in individuals under 60, but not

Figure 2: Relationship between BMI and mortality

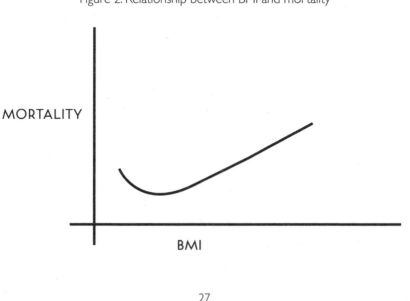

MORTALITY

BMI

27

after this. Other studies have yielded findings that support the idea that, as we age, being technically 'overweight' is not a concern in itself, and may in fact signal superior survival.

For instance, in a study of Japanese men and women aged 65 and older, having an overweight BMI was *not* associated with an enhanced risk of death, and this was even true for men technically classified as obese.[6] In another study, the lowest mortality was found in older Norwegian men and women with BMIs of 25.0–29.9 (overweight) and 25.0–32.4 (overweight/ obese) respectively.[7] Other research found a significantly reduced risk of death in overweight elderly Australians compared to those with 'healthy' BMIs.[8]

Some researchers have suggested that the explanation for enhanced risk of death in those of 'normal' and 'underweight' BMI may be because, when individuals fall ill (e.g. with cancer), they are likely to lose weight. In other words, low weight is not the issue *per se*, it's the illness that causes body weight to be low that then increases risk of death. The evidence for this has been found to be 'weak and inconsistent',[9] leaving us with the distinct possibility that BMIs higher than advised may indeed be better where overall health and survival is concerned.

AS LARGE AS LIFE

One theory that has been put forward to explain why larger BMIs are associated with improved survival in the elderly is that some surplus fat can be used as a store of energy which individuals can draw on in times of need – such as during a critical illness. In one study, researchers assessed the relationship between 'fat mass' (overall levels of fat in the body), and risk of illness and mortality in individuals aged 65 and older.[10] Over time, compared to those with the lowest fat masses, individuals with most fat had a 70 per cent *reduced* risk of mortality. These findings provide support for the idea that decent fat stores can come in handy in later life.

Overall, the evidence suggests that the hazards of being overweight (and possibly even obese) have been overstated. It seems some individuals may have less need to lose weight on health grounds than conventional wisdom dictates. This applies particularly to elderly individuals, as well as those who are of big build and relatively muscular.

What we know for sure is that, when applied to individuals, the BMI is very limited in its usefulness because it tells us nothing about the body's *composition*. Another of its deficiencies, though, is that it fails to discern the *distribution* of any excess fat, too. As we are about to learn, *where* fat is sited in the body has a critical bearing on its likely impact on health.

The Bottom Line

- The BMI tells us nothing about body *composition* and is therefore not a good judge of individual health.

- There is some evidence that BMIs in the 'overweight' category are associated with the best overall health, and this is particularly the case in older individuals.

THE OBESITY PARADOX

Chapter 3

TOXIC WAIST

Human beings come in a variety of shapes and sizes. While some people stockpile fat around their middles, others – particularly women – find their problem areas to be the hips, thighs and buttocks. These differences are not merely cosmetic: research shows that *where* your accumulated fat is to be found gives a big clue as to its likely risks. This chapter explores the importance of the distribution of body fat, as well as how best to assess our weight and monitor fat loss progress over time.

Two of a Kind

A major depot for fat is found under the skin – what is known as 'subcutaneous fat'. However, as this mass of fat expands, there comes a point where the body can start to deposit fat in and around the internal organs of the abdomen. This doesn't sound good, and it's not: this type of fat – termed 'visceral fat' – can have quite harmful effects on the body. Subcutaneous fat, on the other hand, is relatively benign in comparison.

Precisely what it is about visceral fat that is so hazardous is not known for sure, but a big part of the explanation appears to come in the form of the process known as 'inflammation'.

Inflammation is generally a sign that something needs healing within the body. For example, an ingrowing toenail can lead to inflammation – the cardinal signs of which are pain, redness and swelling. Inflammation results from the action of white blood cells (immune system cells) and the release of inflammatory substances. Sometimes, though, inflammation is not localized, but *generalized* throughout the body. This generalized inflammation, sometimes referred to as 'systemic' inflammation, is usually long term (chronic) in nature, and increasing evidence suggests it's a powerful force in the development of conditions such as heart disease and Type 2 diabetes.

Research shows that visceral fat is commonly infiltrated with a form of white blood cells known as 'macrophages'. These cells are normally responsible for fighting pathogens such as bacteria in the body. One theory is that when cells are sufficiently filled with fat, they can burst, which can attract macrophages to 'mop up' the damage. Macrophages, and perhaps other cells, can cause inflammation through the release of substances such as 'nuclear factor kappa-beta' (NF-κβ), 'interleukin-6' (IL-6) and 'tumour necrosis factor-alpha' (TNF-α). You can relax in the lnowledge that these are the most technical terms you're going to have to deal with in the whole of this book.

Apples and Pears

In women of child-bearing age, there is a tendency for fat to accumulate in subcutaneous depots *below* the level of the waist, giving a characteristic pear shape to the body. Men, on the other hand, are more prone to accumulating fat around the middle, and this can lead to a body shape that more resembles an apple (see Figure 3).

However, while men may have more of a predisposition to an expanded waistline, women can undoubtedly suffer, too. Figure 4 shows two women of the same weight (and BMI), one of whom is an 'apple', and the other a 'pear'.

The relevance of different fat distributions becomes clear when we know that apple-shaped individuals are those who tend to

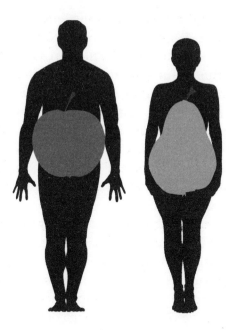

Figure 3: Typical body shapes of 'apples' and 'pears'

Figure 4: Typical 'apple' and 'pear' body shapes in women

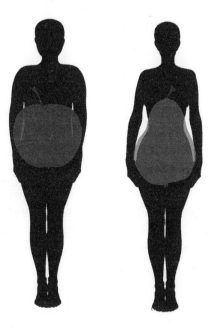

TOXIC WAIST

stash toxic visceral fat: research shows that enlarged waist circumference (often referred to as 'abdominal obesity') is a good marker for visceral fat.[1]

Abdominal obesity is also a key feature of a constellation of health issues termed 'metabolic syndrome'. While the exact definition of metabolic syndrome is not set in stone, it's generally accepted that its diagnosis depends on the presence of abdominal obesity, accompanied by two or more other common features associated with the condition.

For the purposes of diagnosing metabolic syndrome, abdominal obesity is generally defined as a waist circumference of 94 cm (37 inches) or more for men and 80 cm (31.5 inches) for women. The other features that are usually used to establish the diagnosis of metabolic syndrome are:

• Raised levels of blood fats known as triglycerides

Triglycerides are a type of fat found in the bloodstream, high levels of which are associated with an increased risk of heart disease. Triglyceride levels of more than 1.7 mmol/l are generally regarded as elevated where metabolic syndrome is concerned.

• Reduced levels of 'healthy' high density lipoprotein- (HDL-) cholesterol

HDL-cholesterol is a particular form of cholesterol that is associated with a *reduced* risk of heart disease and stroke. Levels of 0.9 mmol/l or less are generally regarded as significant.

• Raised blood pressure

High blood pressure is a risk factor for heart attack and stroke. Blood pressure has a higher (systolic) and lower (diastolic) value. A systolic pressure of more than 130 mmHg and/or diastolic pressure of more than 85 mmHg are generally regarded as significant.

• Raised fasting blood glucose level or previously diagnosed Type 2 diabetes

A fasting blood sugar level of more than 5.6 mmol/l is generally regarded as significant.

If, in addition to an expanded waistline, testing reveals you to have other key features of metabolic syndrome, then taking steps to lose visceral fat and normalize your physiology and biochemistry is likely to be a huge boon for your health. Rest assured: the information and advice in *Escape the Diet Trap* is designed to achieve just this – and more.

FATTY LIVER

Another potential feature of metabolic syndrome is a condition known as 'fatty liver'. Fatty deposition in the liver can be caused by excessive alcohol consumption. However, increasingly doctors are recognizing that fatty liver can be caused by something other than alcohol. In this case, fatty liver is often referred to as 'non-alcohol fatty liver disease' (NAFLD). Once the liver is infiltrated with fat it can become inflamed, resulting in what is termed 'non-alcoholic steatohepatitis' (NASH).

Both NAFLD and NASH can lead to liver damage, fibrosis (a type of scarring) and even full-blown cirrhosis (advanced fibrosis and liver damage). In subsequent chapters, we'll be exploring the nutritional factors that might feed fatty liver, as well as the dietary strategies that may protect against and reverse this condition.

Why Waist?

Bearing in mind that abdominal obesity is associated with visceral fat and metabolic syndrome, it won't come as a surprise that it's also associated with adverse effects on health. In one study, waist circumference was found to be much better than the BMI in predicting the risk of developing Type 2 diabetes.[2] Other evidence links larger waist circumferences with an increased risk of heart disease[3] and overall risk of death.[4]

The superior predictive value of waist circumference over the BMI was highlighted in another study in which the relationship these measurements have with overall mortality was tracked over a 7-year period.[5] For each 5 cm increase in waist circumference, overall risk of death rose by an average of 9 per cent. However, as BMI increased, risk of death actually *fell*. This study provides further evidence for potential advantages of higher BMI values as we age, and points again to the fact that, for optimal health, it makes sense not to carry excess fat in and around the middle.

ARE BIG BELLIES BAD FOR THE BRAIN?

Abdominal obesity seems to be bad for the body, and other research suggests it might be bad news for the brain as well. In one study, the relationship between abdominal obesity and risk of dementia was assessed over a period of more than 30 years.[6] The results showed that individuals with most evidence of abdominal obesity were at an almost threefold increased risk of dementia.

If abdominal obesity increases the risk of dementia, how does it do it?

To begin with, abdominal obesity is associated with an increased risk of cardiovascular disease, including stroke. Multiple, small, strokes in later life can cause parts of the brain to die off, and could clearly compromise brain function (the medical term for this is 'multi-infarct dementia').

Another potential mechanism that might be at play concerns blood sugar balance in the body. Abdominal obesity is associated with metabolic syndrome, which itself is associated with an increased risk of Type 2 diabetes. Raised sugar levels (the cardinal feature of diabetes) can damage proteins in the brain, effectively ageing this organ. It's perhaps no surprise that Type 2 diabetes has been linked with impaired brain function in later life.[7]

Raised levels of sugar can damage particular proteins around the brain that transport cholesterol into this organ.[8] The relevance of this is that cholesterol is a critical constituent of the brain, and performs a number of key functions with regard to its structure and function, including the proper communication between nerve cells.

The evidence suggests that avoiding or reversing abdominal obesity and the imbalances that go with it may help preserve our mental faculties as we age.

Waist circumference is a good indicator of the likely health consequences of any excess fat. It makes sense, therefore, to use waist size as an assessment and monitoring tool. This can be done quite informally by, for instance, observing your ability to tighten your belt by a couple of notches, or finding yourself able to get into a pair of trousers, a dress or a skirt you haven't been able to wear for a while. However, if you want to be more precise about it, you can track your actual waist circumference over time.

It's important that this measurement is taken in the same place and in the same way each time. I advise measuring waist circumference at the level of the belly button, which serves as a useful marker. You need to make sure the tape is horizontal with the ground all the way around.

I recommend taking the measurement on the out-breath. However, slack abdominal muscles will lead to a larger reading than tauter muscle tone here. If your abdominal muscles are not in good shape and you're planning on rectifying this situation with, say, some sit-ups, then your waist circumference may be reduced because of this. To counter this, breathe out but also *tense* your abdominal muscles before you take the measurement.

Waist size is a good measurement, but not a particularly sensitive one in that it will tend not to pick up relatively small improvements that can occur on an almost daily basis. This makes measuring waist size frequently a fairly fruitless exercise. If you want to keep a check on your waist size, I suggest weekly measurements for the first few weeks and monthly thereafter.

Weighing Scales in the Balance

Despite the fact that measuring weight yields precious little useful information and is not much use at tracking fat loss progress *per se*, some of us will find it hard to resist hopping on and off the scales. In their favour, scales are quick and easy to use, and a good set can reveal small improvements that are harder to detect with waist measurements.

I do think it's worth bearing in mind, though, that quite significant fluctuations in weight may occur as a result of things that have little or nothing to do with what you've eaten. For example, on a hot, dry day we can quite easily drop a couple of pounds as a result of dehydration. It's also true that changes in weight may have nothing to do with fluctuations in *fat*. For instance, a healthy but somewhat salty dinner eaten in a restaurant may cause weight to jump up by a pound or two because of water retention. Because of the potential for day-to-day fluctuation, I suggest weighing oneself no more frequently than once a week.

Another word of warning concerns the fact that what the scales register can wield a disproportionate influence over the mental state of some people. Even after a brief period of healthy eating, stalled weight loss or a small gain in weight can cause disappointment and encourage a 'sod it' attitude. If this sounds like you, you might just want to donate your scales to a charity shop.

If you *are* committed to regular weigh-ins, however, I suggest buying a good set of scales. Cheap, spring-loaded scales that were all the rage in the seventies are usually not the most accurate. Electronic scales that are relatively inexpensive will generally do a good job. Put them on a hard, level surface for maximum accuracy.

By now you may be itching to get on and learn how to achieve satisfying, sustainable fat loss and improved health. Before we look at what works, let's explore what *doesn't*. This is not an entirely academic exercise: understanding the reasons why conventional weight-loss strategies fail so consistently will help us escape the trap many of us have unwittingly fallen into.

The Bottom Line

- Fat that accumulates under the skin appears to be relatively benign in terms of its effects on health compared to fat that accumulates in and around the abdominal organs (visceral fat).

- Visceral fat is associated with increased inflammation in the body, as well as an increased risk of chronic diseases, including heart disease and Type 2 diabetes.

- Waist circumference is a good indicator of visceral fat.

- Tracking your waist measurement is a good way to monitor your fat loss progress and the likely health benefits associated with this over time.

Chapter 4

THE BURNING ISSUE

In Chapter 1 we reviewed the evidence which clearly demonstrates that diets don't work. You may well have had personal experience of this phenomenon yourself, and wondered why your body doesn't respond as you're told it should. In this chapter, we're going to explore why conventional approaches to weight loss can fail us in the long term. In particular, we'll consider the impact that cutting back on calories has on the metabolism, and how this may make weight slow to go but quick to return.

Counting on Calories

The calorie principle essentially sees the body as an engine that takes in food (fuel) and converts it into other forms of energy, including movement and heat. Here, in simple terms, is what the calorie principle tells us:

change in body weight = calories consumed minus calories burned.

Let's say that over the course of a day someone burns 2,500 calories through the processes of metabolism and some activity, too, but only consumes 2,000 in the form of food. They have created a 'calorie deficit' of 500 calories, which if repeated each day for a week turns into a total deficit of 3,500 calories – actually, about the same number of calories found in a pound of fat. The calorie principle tells us that by eating 500 calories less each day than the body burns, in a week we expect to lose a pound of fat. Keep up the same game, and there's no reason why, according to theory, that this loss will not continue *ad infinitum*.

This calorie principle is nothing if not simple. The problem is it's also *simplistic*.

One reason for this is that it assumes that, when we restrict calories, the body's metabolism will continue to chug along as before. But is this right? Imagine you're putting two logs on an open fire every hour to keep it going. Now imagine what would happen if you were to put only one log on the fire each hour. Of course, this would cause the fire to burn much less brightly than before. Could the body be like this? In other words, could restricting calories cause a reduction in the metabolic rate that could make it harder for our internal 'fire' to burn food effectively?

The Minnesota Experiment

The metabolic impact that food restriction has on the human body has been the subject of many studies over the last few decades, but none of these compare in scope and importance to a study conducted over 60 years ago known as the 'Minnesota Experiment'. This seminal study was an effort to assess the effects of starvation on the human body, as well as how best to renourish it. The hope was to develop nutritional strategies that would best serve those in Europe and Asia who had been victims of starvation during the Second World War.

Researchers at the University of Minnesota recruited 36 men for the study. They were chosen from a group of 200 applicants on the basis of being the most psychologically and socially well adjusted, motivated and healthy. The study subjects were to live under supervised conditions in which the only food they could eat was that supplied by the researchers and their assistants. The study lasted a total of 56 weeks and was split into distinct phases:

A 'control' period (12 weeks)

During this time the subjects ate a controlled diet designed to maintain them at a stable weight. Under these normal feeding conditions, the men were subjected to a battery of tests to assess physical and mental health.

A 'semi-starvation' period (24 weeks)

During this period the men were fed a low-fat, calorie-reduced diet (about 1,600 calories a day). This phase was designed to determine the physical and psychological impact of 'semi-starvation' on the subjects.

A 'restricted rehabilitation' period (12 weeks)

In this phase, the participants were given more food, but in strictly controlled quantities. The men were divided into four groups, with each group consuming a different amount of food. Calorie allowances varied from 1,900 to 3,900 a day.

An 'unrestricted rehabilitation' period (8 weeks)

For the final rehabilitation period, caloric intake and food content were unrestricted – the men could eat as much as they liked. During this time, food intake was carefully recorded and monitored.

Never before or since has such a comprehensive assessment been made of the physiological and psychological effects of weight loss through caloric restriction and refeeding on human beings. The results of the Minnesota Experiment were published in 1950 as a two-volume set.[1] The data collected from this study were meticulous and voluminous, and this has enabled researchers more latterly to revisit this study and glean important information about the body's response to caloric restriction.

So what does happen to the metabolism when caloric consumption is cut? As the body loses weight we expect a reduction in metabolic rate, as a lighter body will use less energy than the same body at a higher weight.

However, results from the Minnesota Experiment showed that while men lost 20–26 per cent of their weight, actual energy expenditure fell by *almost 40 per cent*. In other words, metabolic rate dropped by an amount significantly in excess of that predicted by weight loss. Other studies have found the same thing.[2,3]

It's clear that when calories are in short supply, the body makes a concerted effort to conserve energy by putting a brake on its metabolism. It can do this through more than one mechanism.[4] For example, quite quickly after caloric restriction, metabolism can be suppressed via signals that come from the nervous system. Another self-preservatory mechanism deployed by the body is to reduce its production of the thyroid hormone known as 'tri-iodothyronine' (also known as 'T3') that maintains the metabolism.[5]

The body can also 'defend' its weight through regulation of another hormone called 'leptin'. This hormone is secreted by fat cells, and one of its chief functions is to stimulate the metabolism. However, as weight falls, so do levels of leptin,[6] with potentially dire consequences for the metabolism.

Yet another mechanism that the body can call into play when food is in short supply is to conserve energy by reducing movement. Studies in animals and humans show that when food is significantly restricted, natural activity level usually falls quite spontaneously.[7,8]

In short, caloric restriction causes a stalling of the body's metabolism and can reduce spontaneous activity, too. What is more, the overall drop in energy expenditure is significantly greater than predicted by changes in weight alone.

As a result of these compensatory mechanisms, it's entirely possible that in the past you may have found yourself struggling to lose weight despite eating sparrow-like portions of food. There's a good chance that you also found yourself plateauing at a weight significantly heavier than your goal and than is healthy for you.

What Next?

Some might argue that there's really no problem here, as long as individuals continue to restrict calorie intake further. However, this approach risks nutritional deficiencies and malnutrition. Plus, of course, eating less and less becomes impractical because it can leave us perpetually hungry. The relevance of this to those seeking to lose weight sustainably is the focus of the next chapter.

SLOW BURN

One of the other potential pitfalls of eating a low-calorie diet is that it could end up being light on essential nutrients. Certain nutrients participate in the reactions that convert food into energy. Could a nutrient-depleted diet stall these processes and cause the metabolism and weight loss to stall?

At least some evidence for this concept comes from a study that assessed the impact of nutritional supplementation on metabolism and body weight.[9] About 100 overweight women were treated with nothing more than a multivitamin and mineral tablet for a period of 6 months. Compared to those taking an inactive placebo, those taking the nutritional supplement saw significant falls in body weight and fat levels. Metabolic rate was also found to be higher, something that was related to more efficient burning of fat.

A calorie-restricted diet could, in theory, lead to nutritional deficiencies that slow the metabolic rate and contribute to the disappointing results seen with these regimes.

The Bottom Line

- During weight loss, metabolism can fall to a degree significantly greater than that predicted by weight loss.

- The body can slow the metabolism though mechanisms that involve the nervous system, and levels of thyroid hormones and leptin.

- Reductions in calorie intake can lead to a spontaneous reduction in activity.

- Nutrient deficiencies may also contribute to slowing of the metabolism during restricted eating.

Chapter 5

THE HUNGER WITHIN

If you've dieted in the past, you'll no doubt be all too familiar with restricted eating and the impact this has on the appetite. The hunger that conscious cutting of calories almost inevitably brings with it can sap the resolve and make healthy changes quite unsustainable. Not only this, but, as we'll see here, making significant cutbacks in our calorie consumption can have quite devastating effects on our physical and mental wellbeing.

Back to Minnesota

The Minnesota Experiment described in the last chapter gave researchers an opportunity to study at close quarters the effect of calorie restriction on hunger, general wellbeing and mood. To recap, during the 'semi-starvation' phase of the study, volunteers ate about 1,600 calories a day. The diet was low in fat and rich in carbohydrate. Both in terms of its quality and quantity, the diet used in the Minnesota Experiment fulfilled the broad requirements of weight-loss diets currently recommended by health professionals.

In this sort of regime, though, the hunger experienced by the men in the Minnesota Experiment was *profound*. Participants were so hungry as to be unhealthily preoccupied with food. Many men confessed to thinking about little else but food, as though it were the most important thing in their lives.

The impact of restricted eating on the psychology of the men was pernicious: depression and emotional distress were common. Sexual interest was drastically reduced and the volunteers showed signs of social withdrawal and isolation. Many men lost all sense of ambition and experienced feelings of inadequacy, and their cultural and academic interests narrowed. They neglected their appearance, became loners and their family relationships suffered. It was reported that they also lost their senses of humour, love and compassion. Their obsession with food led them to think, talk and read about it constantly. Some consumed vast amounts of coffee and tea, or chewed gum incessantly.

On top of all this, the men were often afflicted by physical symptoms, too. Many men complained of feeling cold and tired, as well as having difficulty with concentration and impaired judgement. Dizzy spells, visual disturbances, ringing in the ears, 'neurological' symptoms (such as pins and needles in the arms or legs), insomnia, hair loss and dryness and thinning of the skin were also noted.

And just to remind ourselves, all this misery and suffering was the result of eating just the sort of weight-loss diet recommended by health professionals to this day.

Famine Then Feast

You may recall that, in the final phase of the Minnesota Experiment, men were allowed to eat as much as they liked. Left to their own devices, they ate huge quantities of food, consuming an average of more than 4,000 calories a day for several weeks. Once food was unrestricted, there was a very strong drive to overeat.

One interpretation of this overeating (technically termed 'hyperphagia') is that it's caused by gluttony – a *psychological* response to having had food restricted for so long. Another way to look at it, though, is as a natural reaction driven by processes in the body designed to regain lost weight.

Analysis of the data from the Minnesota Experiment reveals that the extreme eating exhibited by men once the shackles were off was directly related to the extent of their weight loss: the more weight men had lost, the more they ate once eating was unrestricted. As body weight increased, so food intake gradually decreased. Crucially, though, by the time eating returned to normal, fat levels were *75 per cent higher* than they were at the start of the study.

This finding raises the possibility that conventional diets not only do not work, but in fact may be *worse* than doing nothing in the long term.

Hunger Hormone

What is it that causes the rampant hunger so often induced by conventional dieting and the overeating that may ensue? Our drive to eat is not solely determined by how much food we have in our stomach, but is also influenced by hormones that signal to the body how well stocked it is with fat. One of the key hormones here is leptin, mentioned in the last chapter with respect to its metabolism-boosting effects. Another function of leptin is to *suppress the appetite.* As weight is lost and leptin levels fall, hunger becomes heightened, driving us to eat more.

IS CALORIE COUNTING FATTENING?

One of the potential challenges associated with conventional dieting is that it usually requires individuals to keep track of and control the calories they consume. This does not just soak up time and mental energy, it can be *stressful,* too. Restriction of food intake and calorie counting have both been shown to increase levels of the stress hormone cortisol.[1]

This may have special significance for those seeking to lose weight, as cortisol predisposes to fatty accumulation, particularly around the middle. One of cortisol's effects is to impair the function of insulin, which may lead to what is known as 'insulin resistance'. This state, described in detail in Chapter 9 (Inflammatory Arguments), increases the body's propensity to gain weight as well as the risk of diseases including Type 2 diabetes. Some researchers have even suggested that high cortisol levels might be *the* key factor in the development of metabolic syndrome.[2]

It seems that another mechanism through which calorie-controlled dieting fails is through an ability to raise cortisol levels in the body.

The effects of leptin and cortisol demonstrate how fatness is, to quite some degree, under *hormonal* control. In the next chapter we'll explore how the standard weight-loss diet – high in carbohydrate and low in fat – can induce a key hormonal state that is quite counter-productive where healthy weight loss is concerned.

The Bottom Line

- The hunger induced by conscious restriction of food intake can make weight loss quite unsustainable.

- Conscious caloric restriction can have very negative consequences for psychological and general wellbeing.

- Hunger is controlled by a variety of mechanisms, including the action of the hormone leptin.

- Calorie-controlled dieting may hamper weight loss and predispose to illness by raising levels of the hormone cortisol.

Chapter 6

LOW-FAT FALLACY

Conventional wisdom dictates that a key to successful weight loss is to keep the diet low in calories, and a key strategy deployed here is to cut back on *fat*. Fat contains twice as many calories as carbohydrate or protein. It's also called *fat*, of course. These facts do, on the face of it, seem to incriminate fat as something inherently *fattening*. As a result, past attempts at weight loss may well have had you consuming enough skimmed milk and skinless chicken breasts to last you a lifetime.

On the other hand, many individuals will have had the experience of filling up on fat-packed foods such as eggs, cream, cheese and butter on 'low-carb' regimes (such as the Atkins Diet), only to see their own fat melt away. Such experiences should, if nothing else, cause us to question the widely held belief that the fat we put in our mouths is destined to end up in the fat stores within our body.

In this chapter, we're going to delve into the science of obesity. By the end of the chapter you'll realize why low-fat diets may have failed you in the past, and what is most probably causing you to carry more weight than you'd like.

RESEARCH 101

Throughout this book I refer to scientific research, and it makes sense to get clear about the conclusions that can (and can't) be drawn from it from the very start. Research relevant to human health comes in two main forms – so-called 'epidemiological' and 'intervention' studies.

Epidemiological studies:

Epidemiological studies look at *relationships* between things, such as smoking and lung cancer or exercise and heart disease. Such studies can tell us that two things are *associated*, but not that one is necessarily *causing* the other. For example, studies linking to *owning* a television cannot be used to conclude that televisions *cause* heart disease. Here, the association is probably not due to owning the television, *per se*, but other things such as the sedentary nature of *watching* television.

Factors that may queer the pitch in this way are referred to as 'confounding factors', or simply 'confounders'. In some studies, researchers attempt to take account of potential confounding factors when data is analysed. The problem, though, is that this is quite an inexact science, and in the end we still end up with results that cannot prove causality.

Intervention studies:

Causality is best demonstrated with *intervention* studies. These involve exposing individuals to a specific treatment and comparing their outcomes to a 'control' group not exposed to the intervention. For example, if eating a lower saturated fat diet leads to a lower rate of heart disease, this supports the idea that saturated fat causes heart disease. On the other hand, no change in risk suggests that saturated fat is not a risk factor for this condition.

Is Fat *Fattening?*

Some researchers have used epidemiological evidence in an effort to prove that fat is fattening. By way of example, take a look at Figure 5, which comes from a 1998 review.[1] It shows the relationship between the percentage of energy provided by fat in the diet and the percentage of people in a population classified as overweight or obese. Basically, the larger the percentage of the diet that comes from fat, the larger people tend to be.

However, remember that *epidemiological* studies of this nature cannot be used to conclude that fat *causes* obesity. It's perhaps worth bearing in mind that studies that look across different countries like this are especially prone to confounding (see above). This certainly seems to be the case here.

Notice how the countries down to the lower left-hand part of the graph (lower fat intake and lower body mass) such as India and the Philippines are less 'developed' than countries up and to the right (higher fat intake and higher body mass) such as the

Figure 5: Relationship between percentage of calories from fat and percentage of people with BMI of 25 or more in several countries

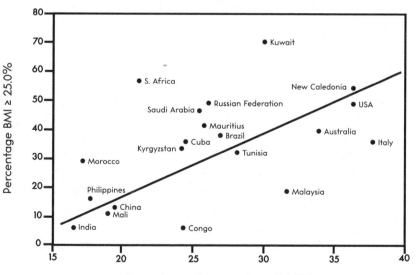

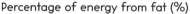

Percentage of energy from fat (%)

LOW-FAT FALLACY

USA and Australia. Less developed countries differ from more developed ones in lots of ways, including the total amount of calories consumed each day, something that is closely linked with a country's economic status.

One way of attempting to level the playing field here would be to compare countries of similar economic development. When this is done, the apparent relationship between fat and fatness simply disappears in men.[2] And in women, we find that *higher* fat intakes are associated with *lower* body weight. Other evidence shows that eating more fat is not associated with increased fatness over time.[3]

Body of Evidence

No amount of epidemiological evidence, however good, can settle the debate about whether fat is fattening. What are required here are *intervention* studies. If fat really is fattening, low-fat diets should be effective for weight loss, right?

One way of getting a good overall idea of the effectiveness of a treatment or strategy is to amass several similar studies in the form of what is known as a 'meta-analysis'. One such meta-analysis was performed by the respected international group of researchers known as the Cochrane Collaboration.[4] The researchers were particularly interested in the ability of participants to sustain weight loss over longer periods of time.

In these studies, low-fat diets were pitted against diets that, although restricted in calories, were not explicitly low in fat (so-called 'control' diets). Low-fat diets produced modest transient weight losses, and, after 18 months, weight was the same as it was at the beginning.

Interestingly, the control diets actually outperformed the low-fat ones. The logical conclusion? Low-fat diets are actually *less effective* for weight control than those higher in fat.

This study was withdrawn in 2008, on the basis that it was out of date, and there were no plans to update it. The fact remains, however, that at the time the study was published there was no good evidence that low-fat diets are effective for weight loss. No new evidence has come to light which challenges this either.

Some might argue that while reducing fat intake is ineffective for weight loss, it may, however, be more effective regarding *fat loss* specifically. This question was considered by a major review conducted by researchers at the Harvard School of Public Health in the US.[5] After assessing both epidemiological and intervention studies, its authors concluded that 'diets rich in fat do not appear to be an important cause of body fatness, and that lowering fat in the diet will not be a solution for overweight and obesity.'

There's perhaps something counterintuitive about the fact that eating fat is not fattening, and that eating less fat does not lead to us shedding fat of our own. All becomes clear, however, when we understand how fat stores in our body are regulated.

Fat in Flux

If you've been carrying excess fat for some time, you might be tempted to imagine that your fat stores are static or *stuck*. In fact, nothing could be further from the truth, as fat makes its way in and out of the fat cells through the day and night. Fat tissue may seem fixed, but in reality it's in a state of flux.

Some scientists and commentators have suggested that fatness should be considered a product of not caloric excess but a disorder of 'fat accumulation'. One could ask what factors drive fat into the fat cells and helps keep it there. Might there be certain circumstances in which foods stimulate the formation of fat in a way that is somehow distinct from the number of calories they contain? Could some foods, for a given number of calories, be more fattening than others?

Fat is delivered to the fat cells via the bloodstream in the form of what are known as 'triglycerides'. One triglyceride molecule is made up of three molecules of fat (called 'fatty acids'), joined on to a molecule of something known as 'glycerol'. Triglyceride is too big to penetrate the fat cells. It must first be disassembled, allowing its fatty acid constituents to make their way into the fat cells. Once there, fatty acids and glycerol can combine again to form triglycerides, effectively 'fixing' the fat in the fat cell.

Fat can be released again, but for this to happen triglyceride must be broken down into its constituent parts. This process, known as 'lipolysis', allows fat to be discharged back into the bloodstream.

So what is it that regulates the ebb and flow of fat in the fat cells? And, most importantly, what causes more fat to go into fat cells than comes out?

Insulin – the Fat Controller

The regulation of fat stores in the body is complex, but there's no denying that a major player here is the hormone *insulin*. After we eat, insulin is secreted from the pancreas. Insulin's main function is to sweep sugar and other nutrients out of the bloodstream and into the body's cells to be metabolized for energy or stored for later use.

Insulin has effects that have a critical bearing on fat storage. Here are its main effects with regard to this:

• Increased uptake of fat into the fat cells

Insulin activates the enzyme 'lipoprotein lipase' that catalyses the conversion of triglycerides into glycerol and fatty acids. This facilitates the uptake of fat into the fat cells.

• Increased supply of glycerol for the 'fixing' of fat

Insulin also facilitates the uptake of sugar into cells where it can be converted into glycerol (via something known as glycerol-3-phosphate). In combination with fatty acids, glycerol 'fixes' fat in the fat cells.

• Inhibition of fat breakdown and release from the fat cells

Triglyceride in the fat cells is disassembled through the action of an enzyme known as 'hormone-sensitive lipase'. Insulin inhibits this enzyme, and therefore slows fat release from the fat cells (lipolysis).

• Stimulation of fat production

Some fat in the body can be made from sugar through a process known as '*de novo* lipogenesis' in the liver. This process is driven by the enzyme 'acetyl co-A carboxylase', which is activated by insulin.

In short – *insulin is fattening*. And, crucially, *lower levels of insulin* will generally lead to *fat loss*. More on this later.

Now that we know that insulin drives fat accumulation in the body, is it possible to explain the observation that dietary fat does not cause obesity?

It turns out that fat does not directly stimulate insulin secretion, which means that it has limited fattening potential.

A FAT LOT OF GOOD

The impact of fat on insulin levels and fat storage was graphically demonstrated in a study in which individuals were fed, at different times, in two very different ways. On one occasion, study subjects were fasted (other than being given a saline drip) for a total of 84 hours.[6] During this time, insulin levels fell, and the rate of lipolysis (fat breakdown) increased, as evidenced by a rise in levels of free fatty acids in the bloodstream. Essentially, fasting lowered insulin levels which allowed fat cells to give up their fat. No surprises here.

The really interesting part of this study came when the same individuals were 'fed' with an intravenous drip containing little else but fat. The fatty infusion supplied the volunteers with about 2,000 calories a day – the amount calculated to maintain a stable weight.

Just as before, insulin levels fell. The rate of lipolysis and fatty acid levels in the bloodstream increased. What is more, the extent of these changes was the same as during complete fasting.

LOW-FAT FALLACY

In other words, feeding the body pure fat induced a metabolic state in the body that was, to all intents and purposes, the same as the state induced by complete fasting.

Obviously, eating nothing but fat is not to be advised. Nevertheless, this study supports the idea that fat is not inherently fattening, and opens up the possibility that a fat-rich diet may actually assist our weight-loss efforts.

If fat does not stimulate insulin secretion, then what does? The major driver of insulin secretion is actually *carbohydrate*. Sugar is a carbohydrate, and so is starch (as we'll see in Chapter 15, starch *is* sugar). Let's think through the implications of this for a moment …

If you were to adopt a low-fat, high-carbohydrate diet, even if you induce a calorie deficit, you're at the same time basing your diet on foods that actually stimulate the deposition of fat in your fat cells and help keep it there. This might make fat loss painfully slow, or may cause it to stall altogether. Later on, we'll be seeing how a diet that limits carbohydrate, rather than fat, has the potential to unlock this physiological stalemate and get fat flowing out of the fat cells.

NUTS – FATTY BUT NOT FATTENING

Nuts are fatty and pack a lot of calories for their size. Many health professionals advise against their consumption in anything but micro-portions for these reasons. Yet, when researchers have reviewed the impact of nut eating on weight, they've found no evidence for fattening potential. If anything, the opposite is true.[7] Can we explain this using what we now know?

Nuts are generally low in carbohydrate, and will tend not to cause much in the way of insulin secretion. These fundamental facts give them limited fattening potential.

Nuts have others things going for them, too. First of all, they tend to satisfy the appetite effectively, which can put an automatic

ESCAPE THE DIET TRAP

limit on how much of them we eat, and might lead us to eating less of other foods as well. I'll be highlighting the significance of appetite control in later chapters.

Finally, nut eating has been shown to stimulate the metabolism in a similar way to what happens when we burn dry wood on a fire. This effect, known as the 'thermogenic effect of food', will be explored in Chapter 7 (Is a Calorie a Calorie?).

The non-fattening nature of nuts aptly demonstrates how the impact a food has on body weight is determined by much more than the number of calories it contains.

Fat Chance

The last three chapters have delved into some of the fundamental reasons why a calorie-based approach to weight loss is so ineffective. Let's summarize now the potential effects of calorie-restricted, low-fat eating dieting here:

1. Suppression of the metabolism to a greater extent than that predicted by weight loss.

2. Reduced energy expenditure due to spontaneously lowered levels of activity.

3. Nutrient deficiencies that might slow the metabolic rate.

4. Hunger, preoccupation with food and impaired physical and psychological wellbeing.

5. Raised cortisol levels that predispose to fat gain and ill health.

6. A biochemical state that, through the action of insulin, predisposes to the formation and storage of fat in the fat cells.

At the risk of sounding glib, I say 'good luck with that'. The evidence shows, and as you may have found yourself, that conventional dieting in the way usually advised by our governments, health agencies, doctors and dieticians is unlikely to do anything but leave us fat, hungry and miserable.

In Chapters 10 and 11, I'm going to share with you yet more mechanisms through which standard dietary advice for weight loss can further scupper our chances of success, but those listed above will do for now.

PROTEIN, INSULIN AND GLUCAGON

While carbohydrate is the chief stimulus for insulin production in the body, protein causes secretion of this hormone, too. Does this mean that protein has fattening potential? Later, we'll be examining evidence which shows that high-protein diets actually promote weight loss. One explanation for this has to do with the fact that protein is generally more effective for sating the appetite than carbohydrate or fat (more about this in Chapter 8).

However, another of protein's important qualities is that, in addition to stimulating insulin, it provokes the secretion of another hormone, too, by the name of *glucagon*. One of glucagon's effects is to stimulate the conversion of triglyceride in the fat cells to free fatty acids and glycerol, thereby facilitating lipolysis (fat breakdown). Also, unlike insulin, glucagon does not stimulate the uptake of sugar into the body's cells. This helps restrict the amount of glucose available for the production of glycerol required for the 'fixing' of fat in the fat cells.

In other words, while protein increases insulin secretion, the rise in glucagon that comes at the same time mitigates the fat-forming effects of insulin.

Is It Only Calories that Count?

There's a common dictum in weight-loss science that 'a calorie is a calorie' – the basic premise here being that the impact a food has on body weight is utterly determined by the number of calories food contains, and has nothing to do with the *form* these calories come in. However, the differing effects of the three so-called 'macronutrients' – carbohydrate, protein and fat – on key hormones opens up the possibility that they have different fattening potential, too. In the next chapter we'll explore the evidence that suggests a calorie may not be a calorie after all.

The Bottom Line

- Dietary fat is often said to be fattening, fundamentally on the basis that it contains about twice as many calories as both carbohydrate and protein.

- Dietary fat intakes are not strongly linked to body weight, and some evidence links increased fat intake with lower body weight.

- Low-fat diets are ineffective for weight loss.

- Insulin is the key driver of fat accumulation in the body.

- Dietary fat does not stimulate insulin secretion directly, and therefore has limited fattening potential.

- Carbohydrate has the capacity to induce significant insulin secretion, while fat doesn't.

- Protein stimulates the secretion of insulin, but also that of glucagon – mitigating insulin's fat-forming effects.

Chapter 7

IS A CALORIE A CALORIE?

Most health professionals and obesity researchers will tell you that your weight is ultimately determined by the balance of calories going into and coming out of your body, and that the *form* of these calories is irrelevant. On the other hand, you may be aware of claims that certain diets have what is known as a 'metabolic advantage' – weight-loss benefits that cannot be accounted for by calories alone. In this chapter, we're going to look at evidence for the existence of metabolic advantage. Knowing this, as well as the sort of diet that appears to offer it, can assist you in your quest to lose weight.

Against the Law

Those who claim metabolic advantage cannot exist usually do so by invoking the 'laws of thermodynamics'. These laws relate to energy in its various forms, and what happens when one form of energy is converted into another. There are four laws of thermodynamics, and it's the 'first law' that is usually used to dismiss the concept of metabolic advantage.

The first law states that energy can neither be created nor destroyed. In other words, energy can be converted from one form to another, but the *total* amount of energy in the universe remains constant. How might this law apply to weight management?

Suppose someone has stable weight over time. The first law dictates that, in theory, the number of calories consumed by this individual in the form of food is equal to the calories the individual expends during metabolism and activity. In other words, *'calories in = calories out'*. Applying the first law of thermodynamics essentially dismisses any notion that different forms of calorie consumed by an individual can have different effects on weight. In summary: *'a calorie is a calorie'*.

However, the first law of thermodynamics actually refers to what are known as 'closed systems' – ones that can exchange heat and energy with their surroundings, but not *matter*. Is this true for human beings? Actually, no: the human body does indeed exchange matter with its surroundings, principally in the form of the food (matter in) and as waste products such as urine and faeces (matter out). Also, technically speaking, the first law refers to systems in which chemical reactions do not take place. But the human body is essentially a mass of chemical reactions. So, here again, the first law of thermodynamics cannot apply where weight management is concerned.

If we're going to be strictly scientific about things, invoking the first law of thermodynamics to dismiss metabolic advantage is simply a non-starter.

Law and Disorder

One of the other laws of thermodynamics – the 'second law' – does, however, have relevance to weight regulation. The law relates to something known as 'entropy', a word used to describe the tendency for things to become more disordered over time.

One example of entropy is the fact that when one form of energy is converted into another, the process is never 100 per cent efficient. For example, only a proportion of the energy contained in fuel burned in the engine of a car is ultimately converted into that car's motion (some of the energy will be lost, for instance, as

ESCAPE THE DIET TRAP

heat and noise). In the same way, some of the energy the human body takes in the form of food is dissipated as heat. That's not a bad thing, as it helps maintain our body temperature and keeps us alive. Also, the more energy we lose as heat, the less likely we are to store food as unwanted fat.

Is it possible that different types of calories have different propensities to entropy? Could some forms of calories be more likely to be converted into heat (rather than fat) than others? Could eating certain types of food help you lose weight in a way that is distinct from the calories they contain?

One way to test this theory is to measure the effects of food on what is known as the 'thermogenic effect of food', or 'thermogenesis' for short. Essentially, thermogenesis is the heat generated by the body during the processes of digestion and metabolism. The greater the thermogenic effect, the more energy is 'lost' from a food, and less energy is available to make us fat.

Of the three macronutrients, protein is by far the most thermogenic.[1,2] One reason for this has to do with the fact that higher protein diets lead to greater protein 'turnover' in the body. When we eat protein it is broken down into constituents called 'amino acids', which can then be reassembled to form protein. It has been estimated that when amino acids are converted to protein and then back again into amino acids, more than a quarter of the energy originally contained in the amino acids is lost, including as heat.[3] Carbohydrate and fat can also 'cycle' in this way, but the energy dissipated is much less than with protein.

In summary, protein has significantly greater thermogenic effect than carbohydrate or fat, and fewer of the calories it contains will be available for storing as body fat as a result of this.

IS A CALORIE A CALORIE?

HIGH-PROTEIN DIETS EAT UP ENERGY IN ANOTHER WAY, TOO

The body requires about 100 grams of carbohydrate a day, so what happens if carbohydrate intake is insufficient to meet this demand, such as on a low-carbohydrate diet? One way the body can make up the shortfall is by converting the amino acid *alanine* into glucose. This process, known as 'gluconeogenesis', uses up energy. So a high-protein diet in the context of limited carbohydrate intake may offer some metabolic advantage through this process, too.

Getting back to the laws of thermodynamics for a moment, what have we learned?

1. The first law of thermodynamics doesn't apply to the human body and weight management.

2. The second law *does* apply, and actually allows for the possibility of a metabolic advantage.

3. Theoretically, diets with metabolic advantage should be ones that are relatively rich in protein (through greater thermogenesis from the turnover of protein in the body) and low in carbohydrate (by enhancing the energy lost via the making of glucose from protein).

Testing Times

One way to put metabolic advantage to the test is to give diets of different *composition* to a group of people while keeping the total number of calories the same. For example, some might eat a low-fat, high-carb diet, while others eat a diet high in fat and low in carbohydrate. If 'a calorie is a calorie', then the effects of these diets on weight should be the same.

Support for 'a calorie is a calorie' comes in the form of several studies that have demonstrated essentially identical weight loss from diets that differ in terms of composition but contain the same number of calories. However, these studies were usually of brief duration (often 4 weeks or less), the issue here being that they may not have continued long enough for any true difference between diets to be detected.

Also, against this negative evidence we need to put the findings of studies that do provide evidence for metabolic advantage. We're going to review these studies in a moment but, before we do, let's recap on the major effects of carbohydrate, protein and fat in terms of their impact on fat regulation in the body.

Carbohydrate:

Carbohydrate stimulates insulin secretion which:

- Increases the uptake of fat into the fat cells.

- Supplies raw materials (fatty acids and glycerol) necessary for the making and fixing of fat in the fat cells.

- Slows the breakdown and release of fat from the fat cells.

- Stimulates the manufacture of fat from sugar in the liver (*de novo* lipogenesis).

Fat:

Fat does *not* stimulate secretion of insulin which:

- Reduces the uptake of fat into the fat cells.

- Slows the supply of the raw materials necessary for the making and fixing of fat in the fat cells.

- Speeds the breakdown and release of fat from the fat cells (lipolysis).

- Slows the conversion of sugar into fat in the liver.

Protein:

- Stimulates the secretion of insulin, but also of glucagon – mitigating the fat-forming effects of insulin.

- Has potential for 'metabolic advantage' through its effects on thermogenesis.

- May also offer metabolic advantage through energy lost in the conversion of protein to glucose in the context of a low-carbohydrate diet.

Bearing these facts in mind, one might imagine that, for a given number of calories, the most effective diet for weight loss will be one high in fat, moderate in protein and low in carbohydrate.

That's the theory, but is there any evidence for it? There are, in fact, several studies that appear to demonstrate metabolic advantage. The first of these will be described in some detail, as it included more than one type of experiment and several different diets. The remaining studies were simpler in design and will be summarized in the form of a table.

The Kekwick Paper

The first study ever to demonstrate the existence of metabolic advantage was conducted by two British doctors, Alan Kekwick and Gaston Pawan, of the University of London.[4] In this study, 12 obese individuals were fed, at different times, one of three distinct diets. The diet compositions were as follows:

1. 90 per cent of calories coming from carbohydrate.

2. 90 per cent of calories coming from protein.

3. 90 per cent of calories coming from fat.

Each diet provided just 1,000 calories a day, and lasted 5–9 days. These are the average changes in weight recorded for each of the diets:

1. High-carbohydrate diet – no change in weight.

2. High-protein diet – a loss of 0.26 kg/day.

3. High-fat diet – a loss of 0.46 kg/day.

These diets were extreme, but so were their differing effects on weight. On a high-carbohydrate diet of a mere 1,000 calories a day, there was no weight loss. On the other hand, a diet full of fat containing the same number of calories brought brisk weight loss (about a pound a day). The effect of the high-protein diet was somewhere in between.

Taken at face value, these results suggest that if weight loss is the sole goal, the preference should be fat followed by protein followed by carbohydrate. These findings may surprise some, but they're actually entirely in keeping with what we know about the impact of different macronutrients on fat storage as well as their potential for metabolic advantage as summarized earlier in this chapter.

This paper was made even more intriguing by the findings of another experiment conducted with 5 of the original 12 study subjects. These individuals were first placed on a diet in which the percentage of calories contributed by carbohydrate, fat and protein was 47:33:20 respectively. Total calorie intake was 2,000 per day. Over several days, there was no weight loss in any of the subjects.

These individuals were then fed a diet high in fat and protein, and low in carbohydrate. Total calories were *raised* to 2,600 per day. On this diet, *significant weight loss occurred in 4*

IS A CALORIE A CALORIE?

out of the 5 subjects. That's right: when the composition of the diet was changed in favour of fat and protein, weight loss occurred in most of the subjects, even though calorie intake was *raised.*

Doctors Kekwick and Pawan concluded: 'If these observations are correct, there seems to be only one reasonable explanation – namely, that the composition of the diet can alter the expenditure of calories in obese persons, increasing it when fat and protein are given, and decreasing it when carbohydrate is given.'

The remaining studies that appear to demonstrate a metabolic advantage are represented below (Table 2). For each study, data is given for macronutrient composition, recorded calorie intakes, and average weight loss for each of the diets.

STUDY	LOW CARB DIET carb:fat:protein	ALTERNATIVE DIET carb:fat:protein	CALORIES CONSUMED low carbohydrate diet	CALORIES CONSUMED alternative diet	WEIGHT LOST (KG) low carbohydrate diet	WEIGHT LOST (KG) alternative diet
5	7:68:26	23:51:26	1800	1800	16.2	11.9
6	10:70:20	70:10:20	1000	1000	14.0	9.8
7	35:35:30	58:21:21	1200	1200	7.7	4.7
8	25:30:45	58:30:12	calories restricted to 80 per cent of daily energy expenditure	calories restricted to 80 per cent of daily energy expenditure	8.3	6.0
9	8:60:32	56:12:32	1830	1100	9.9	4.1
10	41:29:30	58:26:16	1700	1700	7.2	5.8
11	37:41:22	51:33:16	1630	1576	5.8	1.9
12	30:46:23	53:9:18	1302	1247	4.8	2.0
13	8:63:28	56:23:20	1855	1562	8.0	4.5

Table 2: Summary of studies that appear to demonstrate metabolic advantage

Note: one of the studies (as note 27) in its original form employed three different diets of varying carbohydrate content, but the results of only the two most different diets are presented in the table.

ESCAPE THE DIET TRAP

As you can see, in each of these studies, lower carbohydrate diets higher in protein and/or fat led to greater weight loss than the alternative diet.

Now, it's possible that the prescribed food and food diaries in these studies did not reflect actual intakes, and this explains the results. And we do have some studies that failed to show metabolic advantage that I referred to earlier. However, remember that these negative studies were generally short in duration. In contrast, the majority of positive studies were conducted for much longer (several of them lasted 3–6 months), and therefore stood a better chance of detecting any true difference between diets.

Summing Up

While the evidence regarding metabolic advantage is mixed, the following is true:

- In theory, metabolic advantage could exist and should favour diets higher in fat and protein and lower in carbohydrate.

- When metabolic advantage has been demonstrated, it has been in favour of diets higher in protein and fat and lower in carbohydrate.

- The positive studies have generally been much longer in duration than the negative studies, and were more likely to detect any metabolic advantage that exists.

OF MICE AND MEN

One potential problem with human studies is that we can't be absolutely sure what and how much the participants ate. Even when individuals are holed up in a hospital ward and fed specific foods of known quantity, individuals would have to be under 24-hour surveillance for researchers to know what they ate (and in

IS A CALORIE A CALORIE?

particular if other food was sneaked into their diet). One way round this issue is to study animals. In one study, mice were fed one of four diets:[14]

1. Regular mouse food (chow).

2. A high-fat, high-sugar diet containing the same number of calories as diet 1.

3. Regular mouse food but with calories restricted by a third compared to diet 1.

4. A high-fat, low-carbohydrate diet containing the same number of calories as diet 1.

The mice had their body weights monitored for 9 weeks. Mice eating the regular chow and the high-fat, high-sugar diet (diets 1 and 2) gained weight. The mice eating the calorie-restricted diet (diet 3) lost weight.

What was interesting about this study, though, was that the mice eating the high-fat, low-carbohydrate diet (diet 4) also *lost* weight. This, despite the fact that they ate the same number of calories as the mice eating regular chow and high-fat, high-sugar diets, which *gained* weight. The weight loss seen in these mice was about the same as that seen in the mice which had been given significantly less to eat (diet 3).

This animal study provides further support for the concept that it's not just the number of calories but the form they come in that determine body weight.

On balance, it looks as though there is potential for metabolic advantage and weight-loss benefits to be had from a diet richer in fat and protein and lower in carbohydrate.

However, even if such a diet does *not* have a metabolic advantage, there are other potent reasons for adopting one nonetheless. As I'll show you in later chapters, this sort of diet has the ability to improve markers of disease including blood pressure and blood fat levels.

Moreover, where weight loss is concerned, low-carbohydrate diets have a benefit over high-carb, low-fat ones that dwarfs any metabolic advantage they might have. This has to do with their ability to counteract one of the major reasons diets fail – *hunger*. The next chapter explores this phenomenon.

The Bottom Line

- 'Metabolic advantage' is the idea that certain diets may assist weight loss in a way distinct from the number of calories they contain.

- The first law of thermodynamics is often used to dismiss 'metabolic advantage', but it cannot apply to body-weight regulation.

- The second law of thermodynamics does apply to body-weight management, and allows for the concept of 'metabolic advantage'.

- In theory, 'metabolic advantage' could exist for diets that are rich in protein and fat, but relatively low in carbohydrate.

- Several studies appear to demonstrate 'metabolic advantage', and these favour diets rich in protein and fat and lower in carbohydrate.

Chapter 8

HUNGER NO MORE

Hunger is a major barrier to weight-loss success in the long term. If you're like most people, you may have the temperament to put up with some heightened hunger for a few weeks or even months, but are unlikely to endure feelings of deprivation for any longer. Not only can hunger make sticking with any new regime extremely challenging, it can drive 'overeating' once restriction is relaxed. If your aim is to lose weight easily and sustainably, keeping your appetite well satisfied is of the utmost importance.

Research shows that carbohydrate, protein and fat have differing abilities to keep hunger at bay. Putting an emphasis on truly satisfying foods is fundamental to your weight-loss success in the long term. This chapter shows you how.

Protein – the Taste that Fills

Studies show that, calorie for calorie, not all macronutrients satisfy the appetite to the same degree. The macronutrient that, pound for pound, punches hardest in terms of appetite control turns out to be *protein*.[1] Eating a relatively protein-rich meal generally leads to greater satisfaction over the hours after the meal than, say, one rich in carbohydrate. This phenomenon means that a relatively protein-rich diet can help people to naturally eat less but, crucially, without hunger.

PROTEIN EATERS EAT LESS

Most Western countries are experiencing burgeoning rates of obesity, and the US is no exception. A review published in 2011 reveals significant increases in obesity in men and women over the last 3–4 decades.[2] A close look at the data reveals that, while Americans have been eating more over time, this increase has come from additional carbohydrate (not *fat*, as is often claimed or assumed).

But another interesting finding from the data was that the *more protein* people eat, the *less they eat overall*. The researchers calculated that if the percentage of calories from protein were increased from the average of 15 to 25 per cent, caloric intake would fall by about 500 calories a day.

Carb Loading?

Many people are of the mind that carbohydrate-rich foods are filling and satisfying. My experience in practice is that if individuals are feeling a need for such foods to sate them properly, they have probably allowed themselves to get too hungry prior to eating.

Besides, how satisfied we are immediately after a meal is not as important as how we feel a few hours later – it's a food's ability to sate the appetite over extended periods of time that counts. In this regard, the evidence clearly shows that carbohydrate is less satisfying than protein. There's some added complexity here as well, in that carbohydrates that release sugar relatively quickly into the bloodstream are less satisfying than slower releasing ones.

One reason that fast sugar-releasing carbohydrates are not particularly satisfying is that, after a sharp rise in blood sugar, surges of insulin can result that can drive blood sugar levels down to subnormal levels. This state, known as 'hypoglycaemia', can trigger hunger and cravings, particularly for sweet and/or starchy foods. In Chapter 14, we'll be looking at the propensity for commonly eaten carbohydrates to disrupt blood sugar levels, and the relevance this has to weight control and health.

Full of Fat

Studies have found that, for a given number of calories, fat satisfies the appetite more effectively than carbohydrate.[3] One reason for this is that fat stimulates the secretion of the hormone *cholecystokinin*, which slows down the rate at which the stomach empties itself and therefore helps prolong feelings of fullness.

However, it's likely that fat's real power as an appetite suppressant relates to its effect on insulin – or, rather, the fact that it *doesn't stimulate insulin secretion*.

In Chapter 6 (Low-Fat Fallacy) we discussed how a low-fat, high-carbohydrate diet tends to cause relatively high levels of insulin, which will serve to 'lock' fat in the fat cells. Of course, the other side of this coin is that a diet low in carbohydrate and rich in fat will lower insulin levels, allowing the body to give up more readily its fat.

Fat liberated in this way first makes its way into the bloodstream, and can then be taken up by cells (such as muscle cells) where it can be metabolized for energy. As far as your body is concerned, this fat is *food* – just like the fat that a bear uses to sustain itself during hibernation. Let's look at the potential this has for you to eat less *without hunger*.

Imagine you were to lose a couple of pounds of fat over the course of a week eating a diet that lowered insulin levels. Each pound of fat contains about 3,500 calories, so total calorie loss for the week is 7,000 calories. That's 1,000 calories of fat each day that can be burned as fuel and your body doesn't now need to *eat*. Time and again I've seen that when individuals eat a diet that is truly effective for the purposes of fat loss, they *naturally eat less* (often a *lot* less).

Conventional thinking tells us that when someone goes on a diet they are losing weight because they are eating less. But is this the whole story? One could just as well argue that those on a diet that lowers insulin levels are eating less because they're losing weight – the fat they're losing is 'feeding' them and keeping hunger at bay.

SATISFACTION GUARANTEED

The ability of protein-rich, fat-rich, lower carbohydrate diets to sate the appetite was elegantly demonstrated in a study of obese men.[4] On separate occasions, the volunteers ate two different diets, each for a period of a month. Both diets were protein-rich (30 per cent of calories), but differed in terms of the amount of carbohydrate and fat they contained. Here is the carbohydrate:fat:protein make-up for each of the two diets:

1. 35:33:30 (moderate carbohydrate and moderate fat)

2. 4:66:30 (low carbohydrate and high fat)

The test diets were *ad libitum* in nature, which means that the men were allowed to eat as much of them as they liked.

Prior to the consuming of either of the test diets, the men ate a diet designed to maintain a stable weight (about 3,000 calories a day on average). The carbohydrate:fat:protein composition of this diet was 57:30:13. The macronutrient composition of this diet reflects conventional nutritional advice in that it was relatively low in fat and high in carbohydrate.

One of the most notable things about this study was that when men switched to either of the test diets, they ate less than the amount of food calculated to maintain a stable weight. Actually, they ate about 40 per cent fewer calories, despite having no restriction placed on the amount they could eat. This finding supports the idea that relatively protein-rich diets have generally superior appetite-sating properties.

However, differences were noted between the two test diets as well. On the low-carbohydrate, higher-fat diet, hunger levels were lower and this translated into less food being eaten compared to the medium-carbohydrate, lower-fat diet. The average difference in intakes was 167 calories per day.

What this study shows is that emphasizing protein in the diet can lead to a spontaneous reduction in food intake, and this effect is even more potent when the diet is low in carbohydrate and rich in fat.

Fat liberated from the fat cells may help to quell appetite, but as a fuel it can drive up energy levels, too. I have seen very consistently that when individuals adopt a lower carbohydrate diet, in time they usually feel significantly more *energized*. The body can take a little time (generally a few days to 3 weeks) to adapt to this shift in eating, but, once it has, the usual result is high levels of energy and low levels of hunger.

In Chapter 17 (Appetite for Change), we're going to look at other nutritional strategies, as well as some behavioural tricks, for keeping appetite nicely under control and ensuring you don't eat any more than is good for you. Next, though, we're going to review two other factors that can cause weight gain and may be compounded by following conventional weight-loss advice.

ONE MAN'S MEAT ...

Diets rich in protein are sometimes said to pose health risks, including for the heart. The evidence shows that higher protein diets actually reduce blood levels of triglycerides[5,6] that are linked with heightened risk of heart disease.[7] Other evidence links a higher protein intake with a reduced risk of high blood pressure and heart disease.[8]

Some health professionals have expressed the concern that high-protein diets are bad for the kidneys. Yet, two reviews found no evidence of this in individuals with healthy kidney function.[9,10] In one study, no adverse effects on kidney function tests were found with protein intakes of up to 2.8 g/kg of body weight per day (that's *a lot* of protein).[11] Those with known kidney disease may need to limit protein consumption, and should take medical advice about this.

One final concern about protein is its supposed ability to weaken the bones. In fact, protein is a critical raw material for the manufacture of bone, and higher protein intakes are actually associated with a *reduced* risk of bone fracture.[12,13]

The common concerns about protein are simply unfounded.

The Bottom Line

- Protein sates the appetite more effectively than carbohydrate and fat.

- Carbohydrate is not as satisfying as protein and this is particularly the case for carbohydrates that disrupt blood sugar levels.

- Fat can be highly effective at sating the appetite, at least in part because eating it helps facilitate the release of fat from the fat cells, which can then be used to supplement the diet.

- Diets most effective for sating the appetite and bringing a spontaneous reduction in food intake are those that are relatively rich in protein and fat, and restricted in carbohydrate.

Chapter 9

INFLAMMATORY ARGUMENTS

In Chapter 3 (Toxic Waist), we learned how fatty accumulation in and around the internal organs (visceral obesity) can give rise to inflammation. However, there is mounting evidence, too, that inflammation may not only be a consequence of excess fat, but might actually *cause* it as well. This two-way street could cause obesity and its associated problems to be persistent and self-perpetuating. What is more, taking a conventional dietary approach to weight loss feeds these processes, and may well have contributed to your weight issue, despite your best endeavours. It's not all doom and gloom, though, as in this chapter we'll also look at how to combat these issues and escape the diet trap.

Insulin Resistance

Insulin plays a key role in the deposition of fat in the body and, generally speaking, the more of this hormone we secrete the fatter we get. But a potentially complicating factor here is that the more insulin we make over time, the more likely the body is to become resistant to this hormone's effects, a situation known as 'insulin resistance'. This situation is compounded by *inflammation*, as this process can also stop insulin doing its job.

81

One of the chief functions of insulin is to reduce sugar levels by facilitating its passage out of the bloodstream and into the body's cells, so insulin resistance will therefore mean higher blood sugar levels. This forces the body to secrete more insulin in an effort to clear this sugar from the system, which can worsen insulin resistance (and so the cycle goes on). Eventually, the body may become so resistant to insulin that blood sugar levels become chronically (persistently) elevated. The end result is what is known as 'Type 2 diabetes'.

Even before the development of Type 2 diabetes, though, insulin resistance can have destructive effects on weight and wellbeing. It is believed that different tissues may develop differing degrees of insulin resistance, with a tendency for fat cells to retain their sensitivity to insulin, while other tissues and organs, including muscle, the liver and the brain, lose theirs. How might this situation play out?

If fat cells remain relatively sensitive to insulin, then they can continue to take up and store fat. But if the muscle cells become insulin resistant they will not be as able to take up nutrients and can be 'starved' of fuel, leading to fatigue. This may happen to the brain, too, causing problems with mental lethargy and hunger. Insulin resistance can also cause the liver to release sugar, which demands more insulin to be secreted, further exacerbating the situation.

In summary, insulin resistance can lead to:

1. Raised blood sugar levels, partly because of reduced clearance from the bloodstream, but also due to increased release from the liver.

2. Continued taking up and storage of fat in the fat cells.

3. Physical and mental fatigue and hunger because the muscles and brain are starved of fuel.

This picture of someone who is overweight, fatigued and hungry is one I commonly see in practice, and it may resonate with you, too. Insulin resistance and its effects are clearly not a healthy state of affairs, and maintaining and improving 'insulin sensitivity' is an eminently worthwhile goal for those seeking to control their weight and optimize their health. As we'll see in later chapters, exercise can enhance insulin sensitivity. But what about diet?

Taking dietary steps to put less demand on insulin secretion generally makes sense, as does quelling inflammation in the body. At the end of the chapter we'll be looking at what sort of diet improves matters on both these counts. Before that, we're going to explore another mechanism through which inflammation can drive obesity.

Is Obesity 'All in the Mind'?

Imagine someone who eats when they are hungry and stops when they are comfortably full, never counting calories or restricting food, and never thinking about how many calories they burn during exercise either. Yet their weight is rock steady from day to day and year to year. How do they do it? The answer is that their body is somehow regulating its weight quite *automatically*.

For the body to keep its weight stable it has to do a pretty good job of keeping calories in balance. Even if it allows itself to overshoot the mark by a mere 50 calories a day, this would theoretically turn into five additional pounds of fat over the course of just a year.

Another way to look at this is to see your excess weight as a product of your body's self-regulatory systems gone awry.

One mechanism that may well have relevance to you here concerns the hormone *leptin*. We discussed leptin in Chapters 4 and 5, where we learned about its ability to sate the appetite and stimulate the metabolism. Leptin has these effects through its action on a part of the brain known as the 'hypothalamus' – which itself plays a key role in regulating metabolism and appetite.

In the normal course of events, as we put on weight our fat cells increase the amount of leptin they produce, and this results in our eating less and the stimulation of our metabolism to burn off some of our excess fat. As fats stores diminish, leptin levels come down, causing us to eat a bit more and burn a bit less fat.

Some scientists have theorized that, as long as leptin does its job, there's no need for individuals to consciously control weight. Those individuals who maintain a stable and healthy weight without any conscious effort probably have, among other things, well-functioning leptin.

In recent years, there has been growing recognition of what is termed 'leptin resistance'. Here, leptin effects are muted, and the end result can be a sluggish metabolism and heightened hunger – not ideal if you're seeking to attain and maintain a healthy weight. Just as with insulin resistance, *inflammation* impairs leptin's ability to do its job.

What Not to Eat

Inflammation has a role in both insulin resistance and leptin resistance, and fatigue, hunger and weight gain are the result. What dietary characteristics might play a role here?

One major cause of inflammation is spikes in blood sugar levels. Carbohydrates that are most disruptive to blood sugar levels are the most damaging in this respect. In Chapter 11, we're going to be exploring the relative sugar release of commonly eaten carbohydrate foods and the relevance this has to weight and health. I will tell you now, though, that many of the most disruptive and problematic foods include supposedly healthy starchy staples such as bread, potatoes, rice, pasta and breakfast cereals.

These foods also tend to raise levels of triglycerides in the bloodstream. The relevance of this is that triglycerides may impair the transportation of leptin into the brain, which can contribute to a problem with leptin functioning.

Doing Damage

In Chapter 6 (Low-Fat Fallacy), I listed six fundamental reasons why calorie-restricted, low-fat diets are unlikely to bring lasting fat-loss success, and may even be counterproductive in this respect. The limited appetite-sating nature of such a diet, and its potential impact on the functioning of insulin and leptin, gives us yet more reasons to avoid these sorts of diet if healthy fat loss is our aim.

Here's an updated list of the effects of traditional weight-loss diets:

1. Suppression of the metabolism to a greater extent than that predicted by weight loss.

2. Reduced energy expenditure because of spontaneously lowered levels of activity.

3. Nutrient deficiencies that might slow the metabolic rate.

4. Hunger, preoccupation with food and impaired physical and psychological wellbeing.

5. Raised cortisol levels that predispose to fat gain and ill health.

6. A biochemical state that, through the action of insulin, predisposes to the formation and storage of fat in the fat cells.

7. Limited ability to sate the appetite properly, and a risk of enhanced hunger and food cravings as a result of blood sugar disruption.

8. Increased insulin resistance, which can lead to hunger, fatigue, raised insulin levels and further fat deposition.

9. Impaired leptin functioning as a result of inflammation, leading to lower metabolism and heightened hunger.

10. Reduced leptin functioning as a result of impaired transport into the brain.

These mechanisms collectively represent the 'diet trap' that you may have fallen into in the past. More importantly, though, what can you do to get out of it?

Escaping the Diet Trap

If a calorie-controlled, low-fat and carbohydrate-rich diet spells disaster in the long term for weight loss, it stands to reason that a higher fat, lower carbohydrate diet in all likelihood offers the perfect antidote.

Remember, a lower carbohydrate diet will lead to generally lower insulin levels and help stimulate 'lipolysis'. Fat given up by fat cells can be used as 'food', generating abundant energy and quelling hunger at the same time.

Less carbohydrate will mean fewer blood sugar spikes, less inflammation and lower triglyceride levels, too. This will help improve sensitivity to both insulin resistance and leptin, which will in all probability lower insulin levels and assist fat loss, while also improving energy, stimulating the metabolism and further suppressing hunger.

With the cells being adequately fuelled through a combination of food and fat from the fat cells, the body will not sense it's 'starving', and will be less inclined to put a brake on its metabolism.

And all of this, remember, should be possible without any conscious restriction of calories or portion control.

Chapters 18–20 will provide you with the practical knowledge and tools you need to integrate this sort of diet into your life with a minimum of fuss. In the next chapter, though, we're going to see what research tells us about 'low-carb' diets, and how these perform compared to traditional diets restricted in calories and fat.

The Bottom Line

- Insulin resistance is a common feature in obesity and Type 2 diabetes.

- Insulin resistance is more likely if the diet is rich in foods that provoke the greatest insulin secretion.

- Insulin resistance is also associated with inflammation.

- Inflammation in the brain may predispose to obesity by impairing the function of leptin.

- Leptin may also fail to function properly if it does not get proper access to the brain as a result of raised levels of triglycerides.

- Carbohydrates that disrupt blood sugar levels provoke inflammation and also raise triglyceride levels.

- Low-carbohydrate diets should improve insulin sensitivity and leptin functioning, and assist weight loss without hunger.

Chapter 10

DIETS ON TRIAL

In previous chapters we've looked at a range of reasons why low-fat, calorie-restricted diets, with the hunger and restriction that come with them, are unlikely to bring satisfying, sustained weight loss. On the other hand, we've seen how a diet relatively rich in fat and protein, and unrestricted in calories, might counter some of the problems associated with conventional diets, and deliver better weight-loss results. Now that we've theorised about the relative merits of these two different diets, let's see how they perform when pitted against each other.

Testing Times

There are now more than a dozen studies in which 'low-carb' and low-fat diets have been compared head-to-head. In these studies, those on a low-fat diet have been asked to restrict calories (typically, 500 calories less each day than the amount required to maintain a stable weight). On the other hand, those on the low-carbohydrate diet were generally allowed to eat *freely* (so-called *ad libitum* diets). Initial carbohydrate intake in these studies was generally set low (20 or 30 g of carbohydrate a day), though in many of the studies gradual reintroduction of carbohydrate was allowed over time.

Table 3 summarizes relevant studies since the year 2000. The table includes the duration of the study, as well as average weight losses with each of the two diets. Whether the result was statistically significant or not (i.e. whether it was likely to be a real difference or more likely down to chance) is also indicated.

STUDY	DURATION (MONTHS)	WEIGHT LOSS ON LOW CARB	WEIGHT LOSS ON LOW FAT CAL	STATISTICALLY SIGNIFICANT?
1	3	-9.9 kg	-4.1 kg	yes
2	6	-7.6 kg	-3.9 kg	yes
3	6	-5.8 kg	-1.9 kg	yes
4	12	-4.4% of body weight	-2.5% of body weight	no
5	12	-5.1 kg	-3.1 kg	no
6	12	-4.1 kg	-2.9 kg	no
7	5.5	-12.9% of body weight	-6.7% of body weight	yes
8	12	-4.8 kg	-3.3 kg	no
9	12	-4.7 kg	-2.2 kg	yes
10	24	-4.7 kg	-2.9 kg	yes
11	12	-14.5 kg	-11.5 kg	no
12	12	-5.8 kg	-4.3 kg	no
13	12	-14.9 kg	-11.5 kg	no

Table 3: Summary of low-fat v low-carbohydrate studies

One fundamental issue with studies of this nature concerns what is known as 'compliance'. It's one thing researchers telling people what to eat, but whether they follow this advice can be another thing entirely. Compliance is generally good in the short term, but tends to wane over time. As a result, even if two approaches do have generally different effects, the results seen with them tend to converge over time. This is not a reason to dismiss what the research shows, but we should at least bear it in mind when judging study results, particularly longer term ones.

This caveat aside, let's summarize the study results:

1. Statistically significant enhanced weight loss was seen in low-carbohydrate groups in trials of shorter duration (3–6 months) and two long-term trials.

2. Of the trials lasting a year or more, two showed statistically significant results favouring the low-carbohydrate diet.

3. *All* of the trials produced results favouring the low-carbohydrate diet.

Average weight loss in the low-carbohydrate group was 7.6 kg compared to 4.7 kg in those eating the restricted diet. Remember, though, the low-fat dieters had to consciously control how much they ate, while the low-carb eaters could consume as much as they liked. Even though their eating was completely unrestricted, overall they ended up losing 62 per cent more weight than their calorie-controlled counterparts.

Taken as a whole, the research shows that low-carbohydrate diets are significantly more effective for weight loss than calorie-restricted, low-fat ones.

Despite the overall benefits of these diets for weight loss, some are sceptical of them because of their purported impact on health. You may be familiar, for instance, with the idea that limiting carbohydrate-rich grain foods in the diet means that we will somehow miss out on essential nutrients. And what about all that saturated fat and cholesterol in the meat, eggs and butter such diets can include in quantity? Surely that can't be good for the heart?

Subsequent chapters will explore the research relevant to these and other issues. Before that, though, we're going to look for insight into the best diet for us now by going back to our nutritional past.

The Bottom Line

- In studies, low-carbohydrate diets in which individuals can eat as much as they like consistently outperform low-fat, calorie-restricted ones for weight loss.

Chapter 11

THE PRIMAL PRINCIPLE

There's no shortage of opinion about what we should and shouldn't eat; the trouble is that so much of it is conflicting, confusing or contradictory. This book has already explored one example of this, in the form of arguments for and against low-fat and low-carbohydrate diets for weight loss. Other examples include the effect artificial sweeteners have on weight and whether margarine or butter is genuinely better for our health.

Later on in *Escape the Diet Trap*, we'll be settling these and other dietary disputes once and for all using up-to-date research. But leaving the science aside for a moment, what does *common sense* tell us about which foods really are the best to eat?

One strong line of argument here is that the healthiest diet for us will be one based on the foods we've been eating the longest during our time on earth. There are the foods we *evolved* to eat, after all, and are therefore those that we're best adapted to and will serve our health needs the best. Relative nutritional newcomers, on the other hand, are likely to create a 'mismatch' with our ancient physiology and will more likely lead to ill health and disease.

In this chapter, we're going to take a look at our evolutionary path and what we ate along the way. In subsequent chapters, we'll see whether the common sense of 'primal eating' is matched by the findings of relevant scientific research.

What on Earth Did We Eat?

It is generally accepted in scientific circles that the species we call man is a distant descendant of the great apes. Genetically, we humans are most closely related to chimpanzees, and while there is some truth in the stereotypical image of these animals chomping on bananas, it is also true that this primate supplements its diet with animal foods such as meat from hunting,[1,2] insects and eggs. In other words, the animal widely regarded as our original evolutionary ancestor is very much an *omnivore*.

It is believed that our first truly 'human' ancestors emerged about two and a half million years ago in Africa. By about 1.7 million years ago our predecessors had made their way into colder regions lacking much in the way of edible vegetation. This would have made meat eating a necessity for survival. Further evidence for meat eating comes from patterns of wear and tear in the teeth of our earliest ancestors,[3] as well as the finding of stone tools and bones scored by cut marks which indicate that butchering of meat was going on some 2 million years ago.[4]

Around 900,000 years ago, the earth experienced considerable cooling, something that would have made our ancestors quite dependent on hunting for survival.[5] Archaeological remains dating back some 400,000 years also provide evidence for a distinctly omnivorous diet.[6] More direct evidence for our evolutionary diet comes from the chemical analysis of tooth enamel and bone, which reveals that from 30,000 to 13,000 years ago our diet was very rich in protein derived from meat and fish.[7-9]

It was only about 10,000 years ago – very recently in evolutionary terms – that our ancestors began to flirt with agriculture and the consumption of grain.[10,11] The keeping and rearing of animals, and therefore the consumption of dairy products, appears to have come about another 5,000 years later.

What this means is that for the vast majority of our time on the planet the human diet was entirely made up of foods that were *hunted* and *gathered*. What constituted a hunter-gatherer's diet would have varied considerably depending on climate and food availability. Some of our ancestors hailing from colder climes, for instance, would have eaten a diet rich in meat and perhaps fish. Those living closer to the equator are likely to have

ENVIRONMENT	PERCENTAGE OF CALORIES FROM PLANT FOODS	PERCENTAGE OF CALORIES FROM HUNTED ANIMAL FOODS	PERCENTAGE OF CALORIES FROM FISHED ANIMAL FOODS
Tundra, northern areas	6 – 15	36 – 45	46 – 55
Northern coniferous forest	16 – 25	26 – 35	46 – 55
Temperate forest mostly mountainous	36 – 45	16 – 25	36 – 45
Desert grasses and shrubs	46 – 55	36 – 45	6 – 15
Temperate grassland	26 – 35	56 – 65	6 – 15
Subtropical bush	36 – 45	26 – 35	26 – 35
Subtropical rainforest	36 – 45	46 – 55	6 – 15
Tropical grassland	46 – 55	26 – 35	16 – 25
Monsoon forest	36 – 45	26 – 35	26 – 35
Tropical rainforest	26 – 35	26 – 35	36 – 45

Table 4: Percentage of calories from plant, hunted and fished foods in hunter-gatherer populations according to environment

THE PRIMAL PRINCIPLE

had more access to plant foods, and perhaps ate relatively less flesh foods as a result.

We can gain some insight into the make-up of our evolutionary diet through analysis of the diets of hunter-gatherer populations from the modern age.[12] Table 4 (see page 95) summarizes data from a total of 229 hunter-gatherer populations.

As expected, the further we get away from the equator and the colder it gets, the greater the reliance on animal foods for survival. Taken as a whole, the research shows:

- Most (73 per cent) populations derived more than 50 per cent of their calorie intake from animal foods.

- In contrast, only 13.5 per cent of populations derived more than 50 per cent of their calories from plant foods.

- Twenty per cent of populations were found to be highly or solely dependent on fished and hunted animal foods.

- In contrast, *no* hunter-gatherer population was found to be entirely or largely dependent on gathered plant foods.

The evidence suggests that, prior to the development of agriculture, on the whole we were reliant on eating animals for survival. The cultivation of grains would have helped us establish a more reliable source of food. This era, sometimes referred to as the 'Neolithic revolution', led to a rapid increase in population numbers, and a way of life that finally culminated in what we know today as civilization.

This turning point in our way of life is often hailed as a huge step forward for civilization, but is it possible that it turned out to be a big step back in terms of our *health*? Bearing in mind the slow pace of genetic adaptation and evolution, could the dietary changes we have seen in the last few thousand years have ushered in a dietary dark age?

Where Did It All Go Wrong?

We can glean valuable information about the health of our ancient ancestors by examining the remains of their bones and teeth. There is evidence, for instance, that the Neolithic age brought with it a significant deterioration in our dental health, with tooth decay becoming much more prevalent.[13] Bones dating from this period also bear the scars of our move to grain eating: this dietary detour promptly brought about a loss in height of some 4–6 inches (12–16 cm).[14]

There are several reasons why the adoption of grain eating might have led to some shrinking in size. It is known, for instance, that grains contain substances known as 'phytates' that impair the absorption of calcium as well as other nutrients. There is also evidence that wholegrain cereals interfere with the metabolism of vitamin D, which has important implications for bone health.[15]

Other evidence for what can happen when we turn our backs on our evolutionary diet comes from an American dentist practising in the early twentieth century by the name of Dr Weston A. Price. Price had noticed that increasing numbers of his adult patients were suffering from chronic and degenerative diseases. He also observed how his younger patients seemed to be more and more afflicted by dental issues including crooked teeth and cavities. Curious about what could be causing such a rapid erosion in health, Price set about seeking an explanation.

Price had read that members of certain native cultures were generally in good health and free from the sorts of problems he was seeing with increasing frequency in his hometown of Cleveland, Ohio. He made it his mission to discover what it was that accounted for the abundant health of these people. He embarked on a 9-year voyage of discovery in which he meticulously documented the health and lifestyle of populations relatively untouched by dietary changes typically brought by civilization. In all, Price studied 14 cultures around the world, in places as diverse as the Swiss Alps, the Scottish islands, the Peruvian Andes, Africa, the Polynesian islands, Australia, New Zealand, northern Canada and the Arctic Circle.

Price documented his observations in his seminal book *Nutrition and Physical Degeneration*, published in 1939. In it, he presented detailed information about the diets of those he studied. There was, not surprisingly, a degree of variation here, which depended on a number of factors including custom and availability of food. While there was variation in the diets of the cultures Price studied, some factors were common to all: *none* of the cultures was vegetarian, and the diets of each were compromised entirely of natural, unprocessed foods.

Given Price's profession, it's perhaps no surprise that he focused on the dental health of those he studied. Tellingly, wherever he went, dental decay was found to be almost non-existent – this despite the fact that the cultures he examined were accustomed to using neither toothbrushes nor toothpaste. Price also noticed that, in addition to healthy teeth and gums, the individuals he studied enjoyed robust health, despite the often challenging conditions in which they lived.

Price also had the opportunity to study indigenous individuals who had very recently adopted more modern eating habits. He noted that when dietary detours of this nature were made, dental decay and ill health were the result.

All Change

Prior to the Neolithic era, foods now commonplace in our diet such as grains and dairy products were simply not eaten. And only in very recent times have we seen the introduction of considerable quantities of refined sugar, vegetable oils and flour-based products that, again, did not pass our lips for the great majority of our evolution.

Here's a summary of the major changes our diet has seen in relatively recent times:

Grains

The cultivation and consumption of grains started only 10,000 years ago, but now foods such as bread, rice, pasta and breakfast cereals account for about a third of the total number of calories we consume.[16] It's not just the quantity of grain we are consuming that might have some relevance to our health, it's *quality*. While the grains we first ate were hardly processed at all, the Industrial Revolution of the eighteenth and nineteenth centuries allowed the refining of grain on a scale never before seen. These processes not only strip grain of many of its nutrients, but also cause it to liberate sugar more quickly into the bloodstream. The relevance of this to health will be explored in Chapter 14 (Grain of Truth).

Dairy products

Dairy product consumption dates back about 5,000 years, though these foods now contribute about 10 per cent of the calories we consume.[16]

Refined sugar

While sugar in, say, fruit and honey, has been in our diet for ever, the same cannot be said for 'refined' sugar extracted from one food (such as sugar beet, sugar cane or corn), then to be added to another foodstuff, such as a soft drink, fruit yoghurt, biscuit or bar of chocolate. One critical difference here is that sugar found naturally in food (known as 'instrinsic' sugar) tends to be released more slowly into the bloodstream than sugar that has been added to a food (known as 'extrinsic' sugar). Refined sugar became commonplace in people's diets after the Industrial Revolution, and now accounts for about 13 per cent of the total calories we consume.[16]

Refined and industrially processed vegetable oils

'Vegetable' oils do not technically come from vegetables, but are extracted from grains (e.g. corn), seeds (e.g. sunflower seeds or rapeseed) or beans (soyabean oil). The Industrial Revolution introduced food-processing techniques that allowed for the mass production of these oils. Thus, it's only relatively recently that we have consumed vegetable oils in processed foods and in quantities that far exceed those possible when consuming the whole foods from which these oils are obtained. In the UK refined vegetable oil consumption is not logged, but it's likely to be similar in quantity to that in the USA, which currently stands at about 18 per cent of total calories consumed.

Alcohol

The consumption of alcohol may be an important part of many cultures around the world, but the evidence suggests that this goes back only about 7,000 years. Currently, alcohol intake accounts for about 6.5 per cent of calorie intake in men and 4 per cent of calories in women.[16] The effects of alcohol consumption on health will be explored in Chapter 19 (Fluid Thinking).

Salt

It is argued that the earliest use of salt as a food additive occurred in China some 8,000 years ago.[17] Currently, intakes in the UK stand at an average of 11.0 g per day for men and more than 8.0 g per day in women. About 10 per cent of the salt we consume as a population is found naturally in food. Another 10 per cent is added during cooking or at the table. The vast majority of the salt we consume actually comes from our consumption of processed foods such as bread, breakfast cereals, cheese, savoury snacks, tinned vegetables, and processed meats such as bacon, ham, sausages and beefburgers.

THE EVOLUTIONARY TIMELINE

One way of getting a good overview of the changing human diet is to imagine the evolution of man spread out over the course of just a year, with the origins of human life starting on 1 January, stretching to the present day at midnight on 31 December.

ESCAPE THE DIET TRAP

According to this, we are exclusive hunter-gatherers until about midnight on 30 December, at which point we add grains to our diet. At about noon on 31 December we start eating dairy products. Refined grains, refined sugar and vegetable oils make their way into the human diet at around 11.15 p.m. on 31 December.

That Was Then, This Is Now

So, what do these changes look like when we put them all together and compare them to our ancient diet? Relative nutritional newcomers such as grains, dairy products, refined sugar and refined vegetable oils contribute *more than 75 per cent* of the calories we consume.

There is no doubt that, as a species, we have *some* capacity to adapt to relatively recent dietary changes. One example of this concerns the digestion of the milk sugar lactose. Lactose is broken down in the gut by the enzyme 'lactase'. Infant humans secrete lactase to digest lactose in their mother's milk. Mostly, though, this ability is lost in early childhood. About 70 per cent of adults in the world simply cannot digest lactose, but the remaining 30 per cent *can*, and these individuals probably represent a genetic adaptation to lactose consumption.

However, there are limits: our capacity to adapt to a changing diet is limited by genetic change that is generally extremely slow to come about. So while we may be able to get away with some recent changes in our diet, having more than three-quarters of our diet come from quite novel foods just can't be a good thing. And it's highly unlikely that such a diet is one on which we can truly *thrive*.

HOW COME WE'RE LIVING LONGER?

If a change from our indigenous diet to a more modern one is so damaging to our health, why are we now living longer than ever before? Before Neolithic times, the average lifespan was estimated to be 35 years for men and 30 years for women. That doesn't compare at all well with, say, the current life expectancies of about 75 and 80 years respectively for men and women in England and Wales.

One explanation for our improved longevity has to do with the fact that our ancient ancestors were at the mercy of factors such as warfare, starvation, extreme climates and animal attack that affect us less now. Also, developments in medicine, hygiene and sanitation have been instrumental in reducing the risk of death due to, say, infectious disease and during childbirth.

As we'll see in subsequent chapters, there is good scientific evidence to support the idea that relatively recent dietary changes pose very real risks for our health. The logical conclusion, therefore, is that our increased life expectancy has not been because of recent changes in our diet, but *in spite of* them.

Back to Basics

We've seen in earlier chapters how diets rich in protein and fat and low in carbohydrate are the most effective for maintaining a healthy weight. If the 'primal' theory of healthy eating is correct, then this sort of dietary make-up would be expected to reflect our evolutionary diet. Data from hunter-gatherer populations allows us to calculate the likely macronutrient make-up of our ancestral diet. Table 5 shows this, alongside the typical composition of the modern-day diet.

MACRONUTRIENT	HUNTER - GATHERER DIET - PERCENTAGE OF TOTAL CALORIES	TYPICAL UK DIET - PERCENTAGE OF TOTAL CALORIES
carbohydrate	22 - 40	46
protein	19 - 35	16
fat	28 - 58	33

Table 5: Percentage of calories from macronutrients in hunter-gatherer and typical UK diets

We can see that, compared to the modern-day intake, a diet reflecting our evolutionary eating contains:

- Much less carbohydrate.

- Significantly more protein.

- Generally more fat.

It's perhaps no coincidence that it is just this sort of diet that has been shown to be most effective for natural weight control. It may be worth reflecting on the fact that obesity is essentially unknown in cultures with an indigenous diet, and without anything in the way of calorie counting, forgoing of fat or portion control.

Primal Eating – the Original and Still the Best?

But what about the effects of a 'primal' diet on *health*? Some aspects of conventional nutritional wisdom and primal theory marry nicely. For example, fruits, vegetables and fish are primal foods *and* have generally healthy reputations. On the other hand, ancient foods, such as meat and eggs, *don't*. More inconsistencies come in the form of relatively contemporary foods such as vegetable oils, grains and dairy products that we're told are wholesome, nutritious and even *essential* to good health.

In the next few chapters we're going to extend our nutritional enquiry beyond weight, to the effects specific foods have on health. Let's see if the common sense of primal eating is matched by the science.

The Bottom Line

- The healthiest diet should theoretically be one based on the foods to which we are best adapted from an evolutionary perspective.

- Evidence from archaeological remains and the chemical analysis of bones and teeth reveal that the eating of meat and animals in general was a feature of our diet throughout our evolution.

- Analysis of the diets of modern hunter-gather populations reveals generally high reliance on animal foods, particularly in colder climates.

- The introduction of grains into the human diet some 10,000 years ago was accompanied by a deterioration in dental health and a substantial decline in height.

- Evidence shows that populations eating a natural, unprocessed diet generally enjoy very robust health and wellbeing.

- Evidence shows that departure from an indigenous diet towards one containing 'Western' foods brings about a deterioration in health.

- Relatively 'new' foods such as grains, dairy products, refined vegetable oils and refined sugar make up more than three-quarters of the modern diet.

- Compared to the modern diet, 'primal' diets are generally richer in protein and fat and lower in carbohydrate.

- The macronutrient make-up of primal diets mirrors the diet found to be most effective for weight control.

Chapter 12

A MATTER OF FAT

It's probably not an overstatement to say that, as a population, we've become fat-phobic. We've been repeatedly warned, for instance, about the propensity for so-called 'saturated' fat to clog up our arteries and precipitate heart attacks and strokes. Dietary cholesterol has been similarly demonized, causing many of us to eschew this, too. As a result, many of us have been persuaded to give over more of our diets to margarine and vegetable oils, which we're assured are much healthier options all round.

However, saturated fat and cholesterol are constituents of primal foods such as meat and eggs, and have been in the diet *forever*. Theoretically, therefore, they should be things that we are well enough adapted to by now. On the other hand, refined and processed fats that are recent additions to the diet might, according to primal theory, be viewed with suspicion.

In this chapter we're going to see whether common beliefs about dietary fat stand up to scrutiny.

The Heart of the Matter

The idea that saturated fat causes heart disease first gained real traction back in the 1970s on the publication of a seminal study by American researcher Ancel Keys.[1] This study purported to show a clear association between the amount of saturated fat consumed and the risk of heart disease in seven countries. It has been cited extensively since its publication as convincing evidence that eating saturated fat causes heart disease, and Keys is credited as being a major architect of the fear of saturated fat that persists to this day.

While Keys' study represented quite a turning point in our beliefs about saturated fat, one of its deficiencies is that it was limited to just seven countries. When a wider view is taken to include data from many other countries, the supposedly strong association between saturated fat and heart disease claimed by Keys simply disappears. Another major weakness was the *epidemiological* nature of the study, meaning that even if it had discovered a truly strong association between saturated fat and heart disease, this evidence would never be enough to prove that this relationship was *causal*.

Moreover, Keys' study was just one study from more than 30 years ago. What have we learned since? In recent times there have been several major reviews of the evidence regarding the role that saturated fat, or fat in general, has in heart disease.

One such review conducted by researchers from Canada's McMaster University in Hamilton, Ontario, found that epidemiological evidence simply does not support a link between saturated fat and heart disease.[2] Another recent study from Oakland Research Institute in California[3] – this one, a meta-analysis of 21 epidemiological studies – again found that saturated fat consumption has no links with heart disease risk.

Yet another comprehensive review of the relevant literature was performed as part of an 'Expert Consultation' held jointly by the World Health Organization (WHO) and Food and Agriculture Organization (FAO) of the US.[4] Again, no association was found between saturated fat and heart disease.

This review also included a meta-analysis of *intervention* studies in which the effects of low-fat diets (these usually target saturated fat specifically) were assessed. Lower fat diets were not found to reduce the risk of either heart attack or risk of death due to heart disease.

The most recent review of the evidence was a 2011 meta-analysis in which the results of 48 studies were pooled.[5] Each of these studies tested the effect of reducing fat and/or modifying its nature in the diet. In general, the study subjects reduced saturated fat intake and/or replaced it at least partially with so-called 'polyunsaturated' fats (e.g. vegetable oils).

The results of this review showed that these interventions did nothing to reduce the risk of death due to cardiovascular disease or the overall risk of death. In studies in which lowering and/or modification of fat was the only intervention, risk of 'cardiovascular events' such as heart disease and stroke was not reduced either. This study, which should have sounded the death knell for the idea that we should be limiting saturated fat in the diet, received no mainstream media coverage.

If eating less saturated fat does not improve health or extend our lives, one might question the point of eating a diet lower in saturated fat? The answer? There isn't one.

Bearing in mind just how often and how vociferously we've been told that saturated fat gums up our arteries, this notion may come as a shock. Yet it is utterly in keeping with the primal principle – saturated fat is a component of red meat and has been part of the human diet for as long as human beings have been around.

In the light of the fact that there never was any convincing evidence that saturated fat caused heart disease, one might ask how this belief has persisted for so long. In the Introduction I mentioned how some dietary myths are promulgated by individuals, industries or organizations which stand to gain from them. Some scientists try to advance their pet theories for professional reasons. Food companies, of course, can drive the sale of margarine and low-fat foods by encouraging phobias about saturated fat.

Bearing in mind what a colossal waste of time and money the bogus war on saturated fat has been, it comes as no surprise that our governments, health agencies and researchers show a certain intransigence on this issue. Using research rather than rhetoric as the basis for their advice would necessitate them admitting that they've been dispensing bogus dietary advice for years. As we'll see later, this advice is not only unlikely to have done us any good, but may in fact have caused considerable harm.

Steak 'n' Eggs

There is no good evidence linking saturated fat with heart disease, but we should not forget that we don't generally consume foodstuffs such as saturated fat in isolation; we eat *food*. So, is eating foods relatively rich in saturated fat such as meat and eggs linked with heart disease?

In one review,[2] consumption of meat was not associated with risk of heart disease. In a more recent meta-analysis of epidemiological studies, no link was found between fresh red meat consumption and risk of heart disease.[6] There was, though, some link between the consumption of *processed* meats such as bacon and sausages and heart disease. These studies don't prove a causal link here, and, even if one did exist, this is unlikely to have anything to do with saturated fat, seeing as fresh red meat contains saturated fat but eating it has no links with heart disease. Further evidence for the vindication of saturated-fat-rich foods comes from studies which fail to find a strong link between egg eating and heart disease.[7-10]

ANOTHER REASON WHY WE NEED TO INTERPRET EPIDEMIOLOGICAL EVIDENCE WITH CAUTION

We know that epidemiological evidence should be interpreted carefully because it tells us only about associations between things, but not about causality. One fundamental reason why this sort of evidence can be very misleading has to do with how people respond to health information and advice.

Let's go back a few decades and imagine that doctors, governments and health agencies start telling us that a certain food is unhealthy and can kill us. Take eggs, for example. When such health warnings are issued, people respond, in broad terms, in one of two ways:

1. they limit their consumption of eggs

2. they ignore the advice and eat as many eggs as they like.

It's fair to say that individuals who fall into the first category are likely to be health-conscious, those in the second less so. Individuals in the second category are more likely, say, to be sedentary and to smoke, for instance.

So, what happens now? We have health-conscious individuals restricting their egg intake for years, while those who take a more relaxed attitude to their health do not. Now imagine we carry out an epidemiological study and find that individuals who eat lots of eggs are at an increased risk of heart disease. Here's the question: is it the eggs that are the problem, or is it the fact that these individuals are not so health-conscious?

Evidence for this phenomenon comes from a study referred to above.[9] Individuals who ate lots of eggs were not, relatively speaking, at increased risk of heart disease. They were, however, at increased risk of death. Yet egg eating has not been linked with any other chronic disease. So, how can eggs be killing people? The most likely answer is they're *not*. The increased risk of death associated with egg eating in this study most probably reflects the fact that enthusiastic egg eaters are, on the whole, generally less health-conscious than those who eschew eggs.

Monounsaturated Fats and Health

'Monounsaturated' fats are found in foods such as nuts, avocado, olives and olive oil. This type of fat enjoys a healthy reputation, on account of evidence linking its consumption with a reduced risk of cardiovascular disease.[2] It's worth bearing in mind that other good sources of monounsaturated fat include meat (about half the fat in beef and lamb is monounsaturated), eggs (it's the predominant fat in eggs) and butter (see below).

Polyunsaturated Fats and Health

So-called 'polyunsaturated' fats come in two main forms: 'omega-6' and 'omega-3' fats. The main omega-6 fatty acid is known as 'linoleic acid', rich sources of which include sunflower, safflower, sesame, corn, walnut and soya oil. Omega-6 fat also comes in the form of what is known as 'arachidonic acid', found in foods such as meat, fish and shellfish.

The major omega-3 fatty acids in the diet come in the form of alpha-linolenic acid (from plant sources such as flaxseed), as well as eicosapentaenoic acid (EPA) and docosahexaenoic acid (DHA) that are found in oily varieties of fish such as mackerel, herring, sardine, trout and salmon, as well as meat from wild and grass-fed animals.

Both omega-6 and omega-3 fats can transform in the body into hormone-like substances known as 'eicosanoids'. Eicosanoids derived from omega-6 fats tend to encourage inflammation, blood vessel constriction and clotting in the body. On the other hand, eicosanoids derived from omega-3 fats tend to have anti-inflammatory, blood vessel-relaxing and blood-thinning effects. Because omega-6 and omega-3 fats have broadly opposing actions within the body, a balance between these fats is vital for optimal health.

A glut of omega-6 fat in the modern-day diet may have important implications for our health, at least in part because it tends to encourage inflammation in the body. Higher omega-6 to omega-3 ratios in the diet are associated with enhanced risk of heart disease and stroke[11] and Type 2 diabetes,[12] as well as inflammatory conditions and autoimmune disease (conditions in which the body's immune system reacts against its own tissues) such as rheumatoid arthritis.[13] High intake of omega-6 fat (in the form of linoleic acid) has also been found to be a risk factor for the inflammatory bowel disease known as 'ulcerative colitis'.[14]

Higher intakes of omega-3, on the other hand, have generally been associated with a reduced risk of chronic diseases, including heart disease.

A major source of omega-6 fats is refined vegetable oils found in foods such as margarine, fast food and processed foods such as biscuits, cakes, pizza and pastries, crisps, pretzels and corn chips. The evidence suggests that the substantial increase in our intake of omega-6 fats is a potent force in the rise of many modern-day maladies. It is estimated that the primal diet contained a ratio of omega-6 to omega-3 fats of about 1–3:1.[15,16] Currently, the omega-6:omega-3 ratio in the typical Western diet is somewhere between 10:1 and 30:1.[17]

Eating less in the way of refined vegetable oils and foods rich in these fats will almost certainly have benefits for health, as will eating more omega-3 fats to balance their effect.

CAN FISH OIL HELP FAT LOSS?

In Chapter 9 we explored the concept that inflammation can drive weight gain, at least in part through its links with impaired functioning of insulin and leptin. Omega-3 fats are anti-inflammatory, so in theory they might help here.

Omega-3 fats have also been found to lower blood levels of triglycerides, which might help leptin gain better access to the brain. This, in theory, might speed up the metabolism and temper appetite. Omega-3 fats have also been found to facilitate the transfer of fat into tiny engines in cells known as 'mitochondria', where they may be burned for energy.

We would expect these effects, collectively, to assist fat loss. In one study, people supplementing with 4 grams of fish oil a day lost

more fat compared to those supplementing with oil rich in
omega-6 fats.[18]

   The evidence as a whole suggests that including oily fish and/or
fish oil supplements might help speed fat loss, and is likely to be
beneficial for general health, too.

Omega-3 and the Brain

Remove all the water from the brain and what's left is mainly fat.
Fat, one could argue, is 'brain food', and one particular fat that
has received attention with regard to this is DHA
(docosahexaenoic acid). In one study, individuals aged 55 and
older with 'age-related cognitive decline' (impaired brain function
but not overt dementia) were treated with 900 mg of DHA or
placebo for just 24 weeks.[19] Those taking the DHA were found to
experience improvements in both learning and memory function.

Partially Hydrogenated and Trans Fats

The increasing amount of omega-6 fats in the diet is not the only
change we have experienced in our fatty intake in recent times.
Another shift has been in our intake of so-called 'partially
hydrogenated' or 'hydrogenated' fats. These fats are
manufactured in factories, through the addition of hydrogen to
vegetable oils using high temperature and pressure.

   The hydrogenation of fats can solidify and stabilize them,
enabling the manufacture of margarine and other foods with long
shelf lives. Bear in mind, though, that these fats are unknown in
nature, and have only been making their way into our mouths in
significant amounts for a few decades.

   Evolutionary theory would suggest that foods containing
partially hydrogenated fats would not make particularly good
choices from a health perspective. In the last decade or so,
scientists have focused their attention on the health effects of a
particular type of partially hydrogenated fats known as 'trans
fatty acid', or 'trans fats'. These fats are not only chemically

ESCAPE THE DIET TRAP

changed, but have also undergone an unnatural alteration in *shape*. The research links industrially produced trans fats with wide-ranging conditions including heart disease,[20–23] cancers of the breast and colon[24] and Type 2 diabetes.[25,26]

What About Trans Fats Found Naturally in the Diet?

Trans fats can be found in small quantities in natural foods such as butter. Are these naturally occurring fats as toxic to health as those that come out of a factory? Industrially produced trans fats have different chemical structures from naturally occurring ones: the former are predominantly monounsaturated trans fats of which something known as 'elaidic acid' is a major component, while the latter are found mainly in the form of different fats known as 'trans vaccenic acid' and 'conjugated linoleic acids'. Do these differences reflect on their impact on health? While industrially produced trans fats have strong links with heart disease, naturally occurring ones do not.[27,28]

TRANS FATS AND WEIGHT

To date, there are no studies that have assessed the impact of trans-fat eating on weight in humans, but we have the next best thing in the form of research conducted in primates.[29] Here, one group of monkeys was fed a diet which contained 8 per cent of calories from industrially produced trans fat. In another group of monkeys, these trans-fat calories were replaced with naturally occurring monounsaturated fat. All monkeys in the study were fed the same number or calories each day for a total of 6 years.

At the end of the study, monkeys fed trans fat gained more than 7 per cent in body weight, compared to less than 2 per cent of the monkeys fed monounsaturated fat. Also, the monkeys fed trans fat tended to accumulate their weight in and around the abdomen – precisely the form of weight gain that we know is most strongly linked with conditions such as heart disease and diabetes.

This study provides further evidence of the perils of industrially produced trans fats, and should remind us that the *form* calories come in can have a profound influence on the effect they have on weight and health.

IS MARGARINE REALLY BETTER THAN BUTTER?

For some decades now, margarine has been marketed as a 'healthy alternative' to butter. Initially margarine was sold to us on the basis that, compared to butter, it is lower in saturated fat. This selling proposition is obviously based on the assumption that saturated fat is bad for health. As we now know, there's no good evidence for this.

Another claim for margarine is that it is rich in 'polyunsaturates'. But the polyunsaturated fats found in margarine are generally of the omega-6 type that most of us should, if anything, be cutting back on.

More recently, some margarines have been vigorously promoted on the basis that they help to reduce levels of cholesterol in the bloodstream. In the next chapter I'll reveal why this quality is of dubious benefit, to say the least. I'll also be sharing with you worrying evidence regarding cholesterol-reducing compounds called 'phytosterols' that are added to some margarines and other 'functional foods'.

Other reasons to be suspicious of margarine relate to its highly processed and chemicalized nature. The vegetable oils that are the basic ingredient of margarine are usually extracted using heat, pressure and chemical solvents that can damage them and also impart unhealthy properties to them. The resultant oil is then treated with sodium hydroxide to neutralize unstable fats in the oil that may cause spoilage. After this, the oil is bleached, filtered and steam-treated to produce what is essentially a colourless, flavourless liquid.

To convert this into margarine, this oil is subjected to hydrogenation (see above) or 'interesterification' (which involves the use of high temperature and pressure, along with enzymes or acids, to harden the oil). Both hydrogenation and interesterification lead to the formation of unnatural fats. After this, the solidified fat is blended with other fats, which may be of vegetable or animal origin.

We're not done yet: the product now needs colouring and flavouring (using yet more chemicals), as well as emulsifying agents to stop it separating. And, finally, the end result is extruded into a plastic tub, and sold to us as something healthy. *Really?*

Margarine's very nature is, obviously, very *alien to nature*. Butter, in comparison, is a quite natural food. It may not be a 'primal' food, as such, but its constituents (primarily saturated and monounsaturated fat) have been in the diet *forever*. So what does the research show regarding the impact of margarine and butter on health? Unfortunately, we only have epidemiological studies to go on, but their findings are nonetheless revealing.

One study in men found that while butter consumption was not associated with heart disease risk, that of margarine *was*.[30] In the long term, for each teaspoon of margarine consumed each day, risk of heart disease was found to be *raised* by 10 per cent. Other evidence links margarine consumption with a heightened risk of heart disease.[31]

Again, epidemiological evidence of this nature cannot be used to prove margarine *causes* heart disease. However, this evidence is incriminating when we consider that, generally speaking, margarine consumers tend to be more health-conscious than those who eat butter. By rights, these individuals would be expected to have a lower risk of heart disease compared to less health-conscious butter eaters.

The evidence from the scientific literature points strongly to these facts:

1. Fats found naturally in the diet (including saturated fat) pose no threats to health and often have health-giving properties.

2. Industrially processed fats should be avoided (including refined grain and seed oils).

Despite the lack of incriminating evidence regarding saturated fat's role in disease, some continue to warn us of its perils. A central theme here is that saturated fat can raise blood cholesterol levels, and this will lead to an increased risk of heart disease. However, if saturated fat has no links with heart disease itself, then its impact on cholesterol is *irrelevant*.

Nevertheless, the fact that the medical profession reminds us constantly of the supposed havoc wreaked on health by raised cholesterol levels makes it difficult to shake off the idea that saturated fat causes heart disease. In the next chapter we're going to see if cholesterol really is the killer it's made out to be.

The Bottom Line

- Saturated fat consumption is not linked with heart disease, and eating less of it has not been shown to have benefits for health.

- Consumption of monounsaturated fat, found in foods such as nuts, avocados, olive oil, meat, eggs and butter, is linked with a reduced risk of heart disease.

- Omega-6 and omega-3 fats have antagonistic actions in the body, and having the correct balance of these fats is important for optimal health.

- An excess of omega-6 over omega-3 fats in the diet encourages inflammation and has links with enhanced risk of chronic diseases including heart disease, Type 2 diabetes and arthritis.

- Omega-3 fats may enhance fat loss through a variety of mechanisms.

- General benefits are to be had from reducing omega-6 intake and increasing omega-3 consumption.

- Industrially produced, partially hydrogenated and 'trans' fats are linked with adverse effects on health including weight gain and heart disease and should be avoided.

- There is no evidence that margarine is healthier than butter, and the evidence points to margarine having toxic effects on health.

Chapter 13

THE QUESTION OF CHOLESTEROL

We are bombarded from various quarters with warnings regarding the waxy blood constituent known as cholesterol, and its ability to fur up our arteries and precipitate heart attacks and strokes. Concerns here have spawned 'solutions' in the form of cholesterol-quelling foods and drugs. We're encouraged to consume these things, with the assurance that they will help us live to a ripe old age.

Leaving its deadly reputation aside for a moment, it is perhaps worth considering that cholesterol is a natural constituent of the body, and a component of critical substances and structures including cell membranes, key hormones, vitamin D and the brain. Does it really make sense that cholesterol has considerable capacity to kill?

Killer Cholesterol?

Much of the evidence used to incriminate cholesterol is epidemiological in nature. Possibly the most seminal research here is known as the 'Framingham Study'.[1] Framingham is a town in Massachusetts, USA. Since 1948, researchers have been monitoring its inhabitants at regular intervals in an effort to elucidate the factors that contribute to heart disease. This has included analysis of the relationship between cholesterol levels and heart disease over time.

One problem with this and other supposedly incriminating research is that it has focused on the relationship between cholesterol on one disease only – heart disease. However, as we discussed in Chapter 2 (The Obesity Paradox), a better judge is the relationship a factor has with overall risk of death.

Interestingly, the Framingham Study revealed no increased risk of death with raised cholesterol levels in those over the age of 50. In fact, many studies have found that, in later life, higher cholesterol levels are not a risk factor for either cardiovascular disease (heart attacks and stroke) or overall risk of death.[2–11]

The Framingham Study turned up another interesting finding that has been for the most part ignored by the medical community: in individuals whose cholesterol levels *fell* over time, risk of death from heart disease and death overall actually *increased*.

How Low Should You Go?

Consistent with this finding is the fact that *low* levels of cholesterol are associated with *enhanced* risk of death, most notably from cancer.[12–15] Some have suggested that low cholesterol is a marker for 'frailty' in the elderly. In other words, low cholesterol *per se* is not the problem; the issue is that when people get old (and are more likely to die), levels of cholesterol in their bloodstream just so happen to fall. Actually, the concept that old age and frailty cause low cholesterol is directly contradicted by evidence that shows an association between lower cholesterol levels and enhanced risk of death occurs in younger people, too.[16]

It has also been suggested that the relationship between low cholesterol and enhanced risk of mortality is the result of 'reverse causality'. The concept here is that chronic disease (such as cancer) can cause lowered cholesterol, rather than the other way round. However, long-term evidence suggests that reverse causality is unlikely to be a significant factor here,[17] leaving us with the possibility that low cholesterol levels might be genuinely bad news for health.

LDL – MORE THAN MEETS THE EYE

Cholesterol in the bloodstream comes in two main forms: 'low density lipoprotein' (LDL) cholesterol and 'high density lipoprotein' (HDL) cholesterol. Conventional wisdom tells us that LDL cholesterol is responsible for accumulation of fat on the inside of our arteries, and is therefore often dubbed 'bad' cholesterol. We're also told that HDL cholesterol is responsible for the transport of cholesterol away from the arteries and, being associated with a reduced risk of heart disease, is therefore dubbed 'good' cholesterol. In recent years, there has been particular emphasis on the 'need' to get LDL levels as low as possible.

A major push regarding this came in 2004, when the National Cholesterol Education Program (NCEP) in the US published its guidelines regarding cholesterol management. While the medical profession has been quick to act on its advice, not all members of the medical community have been so enthusiastic. For example, authors of an independent review of the NCEP's recommendations concluded, '… we found no high-quality clinical evidence to support current treatment goals for [LDL] cholesterol'.[18] The authors went on to question the safety of this practice.

In the UK, official recommendations are for cholesterol levels to be lower than 5.0 mmol/l. Yet *average* cholesterol levels in the UK are about 5.5 mmol/l. So, in effect what we're being told is that a natural and essential body constituent at *normal* levels is causing disease and death. Does this really make sense?

There have been accusations that cholesterol policy has been influenced by the pharmaceutical industry. Support for these concerns comes from the fact that, of the nine members of the NCEP panel, all but one had financial conflicts of interest that were not declared at the time the guidelines were published.

Is Cholesterol Reduction Actually Beneficial?

Much of the justification for cholesterol reduction comes from studies in which the cholesterol-reducing drugs known as 'statins' have been shown to reduce heart disease risk. However, while statins do indeed reduce cholesterol, they have a number of other properties, too, including anti-inflammatory action, as well as an ability to reduce clotting in the blood. Could it be that the statins reduce heart disease risk through mechanisms that have nothing to do with cholesterol?

Support for this concept comes from several lines of evidence, including:

- Statins reduce cardiovascular disease risk in individuals who have 'normal' or even 'low' cholesterol levels.[19]

- Statins substantially reduce the risk of stroke, despite the fact that raised cholesterol is a weak or non-existent risk factor for stroke.[20–22]

- More intensive cholesterol reduction does not necessarily lead to improved outcomes in terms of disease or disease markers.[23]

Also, if cholesterol reduction does indeed have broad benefits for health, we would expect to see positive effects from cholesterol-reducing strategies in terms of overall risk of death. In a meta-analysis of a variety of cholesterol-reducing strategies, including diet and various classes of drugs and diet,[24] only statins were found to reduce mortality. One type of blood fat modifying drug known as 'fibrates' was shown in this meta-analysis to *increase* the risk of death in healthy people.

Since this review, a new cholesterol-reducing drug – ezetimibe – has made its way onto the market. While licensed on account of its effects on cholesterol, to date not one single study has demonstrated that ezetimibe has the capacity to actually reduce the incidence of disease or death.

SPREADING THE RISK

In recent years, particularly strident health claims have been made for margarines that have the capacity to reduce cholesterol. Some of these margarines contain substances known as 'sterols' that can be derived from vegetable oils and wood pulp that block the absorption of cholesterol from the gut and produce modest reductions in blood cholesterol levels.

As we've learned, cholesterol reduction is, in and of itself, of dubious value. But even if cholesterol reduction had been proven to be beneficial to health, does this mean that something that reduces cholesterol is automatically healthy? If arsenic and cyanide were found to be effective cholesterol-reducing agents, would it make sense to recommend that we should swig them back each day?

The critical thing is not the impact a foodstuff or drug has on cholesterol – it's the impact it has on *health*.

The relationship between sterols and health was the subject of a comprehensive review published in 2009.[25] It shows an absence of evidence demonstrating health benefits from consuming sterols. The review did, however, cite several studies in which higher levels of sterols were found to be associated with an *increased* risk of cardiovascular disease. This does not prove that sterols damage blood vessels, but the evidence is suspicious.

Perhaps most worrying, though, is the evidence showing that sterols have the capacity to damage living cells. In one study, exposing rat heart cells to sterols reduced their metabolic activity and growth.[26] The review referred to above cites other evidence in which sterols were found to have the capacity to damage and even kill the cells that line the inside of blood vessels. Sterols have also been found to shorten the lifespan of animals prone to cardiovascular disease. It's difficult to reconcile sterols' healthy image with these frankly toxic effects.

Focusing solely on the impact foods or drugs have on cholesterol levels allows industry to profit from products that have no proven benefits for health, and that may in fact be detrimental in this regard.

Is It Safe?

Much of the idea that we should eat a low-fat, high-carbohydrate diet was based on the belief that consuming saturated fat and cholesterol is bad for the health of our heart and circulation. Yet, not only does this belief have no scientific backing now, it never did.

For the last 30-odd years, our governments, health experts and health agencies have encouraged us to take part in what amounts to a mass experiment that seems to have done nothing to improve our health or to save lives. Worse still, this way of eating was vigorously promoted before we had any idea about its *safety*. As we'll see in the next chapter, there is evidence that the low-fat, high-carbohydrate diet we've had rammed down our throats poses genuine threats to health.

The Bottom Line

- Elevated cholesterol levels do not appear to be a significant risk factor for cardiovascular disease or overall risk of death in later life.

- Low cholesterol levels are associated with higher risk of death.

- There is good reason to believe that the cardiovascular disease-reducing effects of statins are not due to their cholesterol-reducing effects.

- The evidence, taken as a whole, does not support the concept that cholesterol reduction has broad benefits for health.

- Cholesterol-reducing agents known as 'sterols' do not appear to benefit health, and evidence suggests they have toxic effects on the body.

Chapter 14

GRAIN OF TRUTH

Grain-based foods such as bread, rice, pasta and breakfast cereals are staples in the Western diet, and are promoted on the basis that they provide energy for the body while being naturally low in fat. Wholegrains such as wholemeal bread, certain breakfast cereals and brown rice have the added advantage, we are told, of being rich in fibre and essential nutrients. No wonder, then, that doctors, dieticians and health agencies encourage us to make starchy carbohydrates the cornerstone of our diets.

Earlier, though, we learned how a carbohydrate-rich diet may be counterproductive for weight loss, and may even feed obesity over the long term through a variety of mechanisms. Also, the very fact that grains are, in the grand scheme of things, a very recent addition to the human diet, might cause us to be cautious about their consumption.

In this chapter we're going to explore whether grains really are the staff of life. Let's start by going over some physiology that is critical to the understanding of how carbohydrate-rich foods impact health.

From Starch into Sugar

Grains are rich in starch, which itself is comprised of chains of sugar (glucose) molecules. Once a starchy food is eaten, it must be broken down through digestion into glucose before it can be absorbed through the gut wall and into the bloodstream. This means that whether we eat sugar, starch or a combination of both, blood sugar levels will subsequently rise. In response, a healthy functioning pancreas will secrete insulin, one of the chief functions of which is to reduce blood sugar levels by facilitating its passage into the body's cells.

However, in Chapter 6 (Low-Fat Fallacy), we learned how insulin also stimulates deposition of fat in the body. Here's a reminder of some of insulin's chief effects in this regard:

- Increased uptake of fat into the fat cells.

- Increased supply of glycerol for the 'fixing' of fat in the fat cells.

- Inhibition of fat breakdown and release from the fat cells.

- Stimulation of fat production in the liver.

Insulin is fattening, and because carbohydrate causes insulin secretion it most certainly cannot be eaten with impunity where weight is concerned.

However, not all carbohydrates are created equal: some are more disruptive to blood sugar and insulin levels than others. The extent to which a food raises blood sugar is referred to as its 'glycaemic index', or 'GI'. Pure glucose, a very fast-releasing food indeed, is assigned a GI of 100, against which other foods can be compared. The higher a food's glycaemic index, the more disruptive its effects on blood sugar are, and the more fat-making insulin will tend to be released in response to it.

The fattening potential of high-GI foods was highlighted in an animal study.[1] Here, mice were fed either a low- or high-GI diet, each containing the same number of calories, for a period of 40 weeks. At the end of the study, the mice that had been fed the high-GI diet had, overall, 40 per cent more body fat.

Let's review the GI values of some of the most commonly eaten carbohydrate foods.[2]

	GLYCAEMIC INDEX
bread	
baguette ('French Stick')	95
bagel – white	72
wheat bread – white	70
bread – wholemeal	71
rye bread – wholemeal	58
bread – spelt, wholemeal	63
rye bread – pumpernickel	46
crackers	
rye crispbread	64
cream cracker	65
water cracker	71
rice cake	78
corn chips	63
potato crisps	54
popcorn	72
pasta, rice and related foods	
brown rice	55
basmati rice	58
rice – Arborio (risotto rice)	69
rice – white	64
rice – pearl	25
pasta – corn	78
gnocchi	68
pasta – durum wheat	44
pasta – wholewheat	37
couscous	65
sweet foods	
digestive biscuit	59
croissant	67
crumpet	69
doughnut	76
muffin – bran	60
scone	92
shortbread	64
ice cream	61
low fat yoghurt	27
Mars bar	65
muesli bar	65
Snickers bar	55
honey	55
sucrose (table sugar)	68
beverages	
apple juice (unsweetened)	40
cranberry juice	56
orange juice	50
Gatorade	78
tomato juice	38
Coca Cola	53
Fanta	68
Lucozade	95

Table 6: Glycaemic indices of common carbohydrate foods

GRAIN OF TRUTH

	GLYCAEMIC INDEX
breakfast cereals	
All Bran	42
bran flakes	74
cornflakes	81
muesli	40 – 66
porridge (homemade)	58
porridge (instant)	66
Special K	54 – 84
shredded wheat	75
raisin bran	61
fruit	
apple	38
apple (dried)	29
banana	52
mango	51
grapes	46
kiwi fruit	53
cherries	22
peach	42
pear	38
pineapple	59
plum	39
watermelon	72
figs (dried)	61
apricots (dried)	31
sultanas	60
raisins	64
prunes	29
strawberries	40
legumes (beans, lentils, peas)	
baked beans	48
black-eyed peas	42
butter beans	31
chickpeas	28
hummus	6
kidney beans	28
lentils – green	30
lentils – red	26
peas – dried then boiled	22
peas – boiled	48
vegetables	
peas – boiled	48
parsnips	97
potato – baked	85
potato – boiled	50
potato – new	57
chips (french fries)	75
potato – mashed	74
potato – instant	85
yam	37
carrots – raw	16
carrots – cooked	58
pumpkin	75
beetroot	64

Table 6: Glycaemic indices of common carbohydrate foods

While there is some debate about how GIs should be classified, a decent guide would be to view GIs of 70 or more as 'high', GIs of 50–69 inclusive as 'medium' and GIs of 49 or less as 'low'.

Looking at the list one thing is clear: many starchy carbohydrates we're encouraged to have our fill of turn out to be very disruptive to blood sugar levels. Several of these staples, notably cornflakes, wholemeal bread and baked potatoes, have GIs even higher than table sugar (sucrose). Some are almost as disruptive to glucose levels as consuming, err, pure glucose.

Look closely at the GI list and you will see that some fruit and vegetables, including beetroot, pineapple and watermelon, have quite high GIs, too. Does that mean that these foods are equivalent to those with similar GIs such as corn chips and Mars bars?

Actually, while the GI is an important measure of the nutritional attribute of a food, it's not the sole arbiter of its effects on health. For example, the nutritional value of food is important, too – something we'll be looking at later in the chapter.

How much we eat of a food is also critical. Foods with a relatively high GI will be most disruptive if we eat a lot of them. The eating of disruptive foods matters much less if we consume them in relatively small amounts.

For example, anyone who goes hungry all day only to come home and polish off a plateful or two of pasta is likely to experience considerable disruption in blood sugar and insulin levels. On the other hand, it's highly unlikely that anyone, however famished, is going to find themselves gorging on mounds of beetroot or pineapple.

This concept has spawned another measure known as the 'glycaemic *load*' (GL). This is calculated by multiplying a food's GI by a standard portion of that food. GL values have been found to provide a much better idea of the impact of a food on sugar and insulin levels compared to the GI.[3] One problem with GL values, though, is that they are based on standard portion sizes. In the real world people generally don't eat standard portion sizes. However, it's still worth looking at GL values of specific foods to gauge the likely overall effects on blood sugar and insulin of consuming them.

Here again is a list of common carbohydrate foods with their GI values, this time with their GL values alongside them:

	GLYCAEMIC INDEX	GLYCAEMIC LOAD
bread		
baguette ('French Stick')	95	15
bagel – white	72	25
wheat bread – white	70	10
bread – wholemeal	71	9
rye bread – wholemeal	58	8
bread – spelt, wholemeal	63	12
rye bread – pumpernickel	46	5
crackers		
rye crispbread	64	11
cream cracker	65	11
water cracker	71	13
rice cake	78	17
corn chips	63	17
potato crisps	54	11
popcorn	72	8
pasta, rice and related foods		
brown rice	55	18
basmati rice	58	22
rice – Arborio (risotto rice)	69	36
rice – white	64	23
rice – pearl	25	11
pasta – corn	78	32
gnocchi	68	33
pasta – durum wheat	44	21
pasta – wholewheat	37	16
couscous	65	23
sweet foods		
digestive biscuit	59	10
croissant	67	17
crumpet	69	13
doughnut	76	17
muffin – bran	60	15
scone	92	7
shortbread	64	10
ice cream	61	8
low fat yoghurt	27	7
Mars bar	65	26
muesli bar	65	26
Snickers bar	55	19
honey	55	10
sucrose (table sugar)	68	7 (10g)
beverages		
apple juice (unsweetened)	40	12
cranberry juice	56	16
orange juice	50	13
Gatorade	78	12
tomato juice	38	4
Coca cola	53	14
Fanta	68	23
Lucozade	95	40

	GLYCAEMIC INDEX	GLYCAEMIC LOAD
breakfast cereals		
All Bran	42	8
bran flakes	74	13
cornflakes	81	21
muesli	40 - 66	12
porridge (homemade)	58	13
porridge (instant)	66	17
Special K	54 - 84	11 - 20
shredded wheat	75	15
raisin bran	61	12
fruit		
apple	38	6
apple (dried)	29	10
banana	52	12
mango	51	8
grapes	46	8
kiwi fruit	53	6
cherries	22	3
peach	42	5
pear	38	4
pineapple	59	7
plum	39	5
watermelon	72	4
figs (dried)	61	16
apricots (dried)	31	9
sultanas	60	25
raisins	64	28
prunes	29	10
strawberries	40	1
legumes (beans, lentils, peas)		
baked beans	48	7
black-eyed peas	42	13
butter beans	31	6
chickpeas	28	8
hummus	6	0
kidney beans	28	7
lentils - green	30	5
lentils - red	26	5
peas - dried then boiled	22	2
peas - boiled	48	3
vegetables		
peas - boiled	48	3
parsnips	97	12
potato - baked	85	26
potato - boiled	50	14
potato - new	57	12
chips (french fries)	75	22
potato - mashed	74	15
potato - instant	85	17
yam	37	13
carrots - raw	16	1
carrots - cooked	58	3
pumpkin	75	3
beetroot	64	5

Table 7: Glycaemic indices and glycaemic loads of common carbohydrate foods

GRAIN OF TRUTH

Just as with the GI, what constitutes high or low GL is arbitrary. A rough guide, though, would be to see GLs of 20 or more as 'high', those of 10 or less as 'low', with anything in between being 'medium'.

Looking at GL values we see a different picture emerging from the one painted when judging foods by GI alone. Many of the foods of medium or high GI turn out to have low GLs. Examples include kiwi fruit (GI 53 GL 6), pineapple (GI 59 GL 7), watermelon (GI 72 GL 4), cooked carrots (GI 58 GL 3) and beetroot (GI 64 GL 5). On the other hand, potatoes and many of the grain-based foods with medium or high GI have relatively high GLs, too. Examples include bagels (GI 72 GL 25), white rice (GI 64 GL 23), rice cakes (GI 78 GL 17), cornflakes (GI 81 GL 21), baked potato (GI 85 GL 26) and pasta (GI 44 GL 21).

It's not just the fast sugar-releasing nature of the grain-based foods and potatoes that poses problems for the body, but the fact that they tend to be eaten *in quantity*. Eating less of these foods will help to lower your insulin levels, which in turn will assist *fat loss*, pure and simple.

LOW-GI VERSUS LOW-CARB

There is little doubt, I think, that eating a low-GI diet is healthier and more likely to induce fat loss and other benefits for health than a higher GI one. However, someone eating a low-GI diet could still end up secreting stacks of insulin over time if the diet is rich enough in carbohydrate. Eating a diet low in carbohydrate may therefore be a better choice for those seeking to maximize their fat loss.

The precise definition of a low-carbohydrate diet varies, and some commentators have suggested that diets containing 50–150 g of carbohydrate each day should be viewed as 'low-carb'.[4] Some dietary plans recommend even more carbohydrate restriction, particularly in their early stages. For example, the Atkins Diet has an induction (initial) phase that permits a daily carbohydrate quota of no more than 20 g. Diets that restrict carbohydrate to this extent are generally considered 'very low carbohydrate diets'.

ESCAPE THE DIET TRAP

Very low carbohydrate diets are renowned for their ability to induce what is known as 'ketosis'. This metabolic state is induced when dietary carbohydrate is restricted and the body turns to fat for its primary fuel. Fat can be broken down into ketones, which provide ready fuel for the body, including the brain. Ketones can be excreted from the body via the breath, giving it a faint odour of something like pear drops. Many doctors and dieticians critical of low-carbohydrate eating describe this as 'bad breath'. However, the breath of someone in ketosis is not 'bad', it is just *different*.

Another common criticism of ketosis is that it is an inherently unhealthy state that is damaging to the body. Those who believe this to be the case are confusing ketosis with what is known as 'ketoacidosis', a potentially fatal metabolic state that occurs in uncontrolled Type 1 diabetes. Ketosis is not a disease state, but a natural response that the body employs to generate energy when carbohydrate is in short supply.

I have nothing against ketosis for this very reason, though it should be said that, generally speaking, effective weight loss does not depend on ketosis. The dietary recommendations advocated here may or may not, depending on your food preferences, put you into a state of ketosis. Whether they do or don't is not especially important as, either way, the end result is likely to be weight loss without conscious calorie control or hunger.

Foods of relatively high GI and GL have fattening potential, but their hazards do not end there. Even in the short term, these foods can have adverse effects on health and wellbeing through their impact on blood sugar balance.

High and Lows

Any food that causes a big spike in blood sugar is likely to cause a surge of insulin in response. There's the risk that this can cause blood sugar levels to plunge to sub-normal levels (hypoglycaemia) some time (usually 2–3 hours) later. Ways in which this manifests itself include:

Hunger and Food Cravings

When blood sugar levels dip, the brain can be starved of fuel, which can cause us to feel hungry (even when there's food in the stomach). It's perhaps no surprise that the more disruptive a food is (the higher its GI) the less sating it is.[5] Eating high GI foods may lead to a drop in blood sugar levels that is known to stimulate hunger.[6]

Drops in blood sugar commonly trigger a desire (sometimes overwhelming) to eat sweet foods such as milk chocolate, biscuits or cake. Some people imagine that succumbing to such foods is down to a weak will, lack of self-control or inadequate personality. In reality, the underlying problem is usually *physiological* rather than psychological.

Fatigue

Sugar tends to provide ready fuel for the body and, if supply stalls, so can energy. Blood sugar imbalance can manifest itself as fluctuating energy during the day, with the mid–late afternoon being a common low point.

Mental Fatigue

The brain constitutes only about 2 per cent of our weight, but it uses about 25 per cent of the sugar in the body. In other words, the brain is one sugar-dependent organ. If it's not adequately fuelled, it tends to malfunction. Common symptoms include poor concentration, loss of focus and sleepiness. Ever wondered why the mid–late afternoon can leave you devoid of energy and inspiration? It might have something to do with that sandwich, roll or baguette you ate at lunch.

Mood Problems

Under-fuelling can also cause low mood and depression. Also, though, when blood sugar levels drop, the body activates parts of the nervous system and secretes hormones that turn on the stress response. Anxiety and nervousness can result. Also, in response to low blood sugar, the brain will ramp up its production of a chemical known as 'glutamate', which can cause feelings of agitation and excitability.

Waking in the Night

Low blood sugar can occur in the night (after, say, a dinner comprising pasta, pudding and half a bottle of wine). Typically, blood sugar levels will fall at around 3.30 or 4.00 a.m. Activation of the stress response (see above) does nothing to aid restful sleep. Many individuals will be tripped into wakefulness, and may find it difficult to drop off again, too.

Stabilizing blood sugar levels will help you remain awake during the day, stay asleep during the night, improve your mood and reduce any urge to eat foods you know are not the best for you. A key approach here is cutting back on foods that tend to disrupt blood sugar and insulin. Taking this approach may have benefits for health in the long-term, too, as high GI and GL foods don't just promote weight gain, but are associated with an increased risk of chronic disease.

GL and Insulin Resistance

High GL diets will generally cause high levels of insulin, which in turn increases the risk of developing insulin resistance. In one study, a 15-unit increase in GL dietary value was associated with a more than doubling in risk of insulin resistance.[7]

GL and Diabetes

Insulin resistance is a precursor of the condition Type 2 diabetes. Another factor that may play a part in Type 2 diabetes is 'pancreatic exhaustion' – copious secretion of insulin in the long term can cause the insulin-secreting cells in the pancreas to 'burn out'. In one study, individuals with the diets of highest GL were found to be about two and a half times more likely to develop Type 2 diabetes compared to those who consumed diets of lowest GL.[8] Other evidence also links high GI and/or GL diets with increased diabetes risk.[9–11]

CARBOHYDRATE AND FATTY LIVER

In Chapter 3 (Toxic Waist) mention was made of the condition 'fatty liver', which often comes as part and parcel of the condition 'metabolic syndrome' (the hallmark feature of which is abdominal obesity). In time, fatty liver can lead to fibrosis of this organ and full-blown cirrhosis. Alcohol can be a factor in these problems, but there's increasing recognition that other elements of the diet can also play a role.

Some insight here has come from a study in which a group of healthy men and women were fed two fast-food meals every day for four weeks.[12] Over the course of the study, those on the fast-food regime put on an average of about 6.5 kg in weight, with waist size seeing particular expansion. Fat levels in the liver increased 150 per cent (quite a feat in just four weeks), and there was biochemical evidence of liver damage, too.

Researchers found that the one element of the diet that appeared to have a bearing on liver health was carbohydrate: the higher the amount of carbohydrate there was in the diet, the more evidence of liver damage was seen. This was not the case for dietary fat. One potential explanation for this observation is that carbohydrate drives insulin production, which in turn drives fat production in the liver (*de novo* lipogenesis).

Another reminder of the potentially liver-fattening effects of carbohydrate on the liver concerns the making of goose and duck foie gras. What is it that these animals are fed to turn their livers into almost pure fat? The answer is *grain* (corn).

More importantly, though, does eating a lower carbohydrate diet help clear fat from the liver? You bet it does: in one study, a

ESCAPE THE DIET TRAP

low-carbohydrate diet was found to lead to significant reductions in levels of fat in the liver after just three days.[13]

Is Low-Carbohydrate High-Risk?

It's probably fair to say that low-carbohydrate diets do not enjoy the healthiest of reputations, with a common concern here being that their generally fatty nature will increase the risk of heart disease. One way to gauge the impact of diets is to assess their effects on 'diseases markers' such as blood fat levels and blood pressure. So what happens here when individuals cut back on carbs?

Here's a summary of the metabolic changes usually seen on a low-carbohydrate diet.[14] After each change, I've added in brackets whether the change would *traditionally* be regarded as a good or bad thing from heart disease risk perspective:

- Improved insulin sensitivity (good).

- Reduced blood pressure (good).

- Reduced triglyceride levels (good).

- Higher levels of HDL cholesterol (good).

- Higher levels of LDL cholesterol (bad).

Looking at this from a conventional perspective, low-carbohydrate regimes seem to win out over higher carb ones for almost all disease markers. The one potential fly in the ointment (albeit from a conventional perspective) is the raised level of LDL cholesterol these diets can sometimes induce. As we learned in the last chapter, this is the form of cholesterol said to increase our risk of cardiovascular disease. However, we also saw there how the role that cholesterol has in health is very much open to question. Even if we believe LDL cholesterol poses risks to health, though, there's something else about it that we need to be aware of.

LDL – Size Matters

LDL cholesterol varies in size, ranging from small, dense particles up to much larger, less dense ('fluffy') particles. It has been known for a long time that the size and density of LDL particles has an important bearing on apparent risk of heart disease. What the evidence shows is this: small, dense LDL particles are associated with an increased risk of heart disease, while large, 'fluffy' LDL particles are not.[15]

What effect does diet have on LDL particle size? In one study, individuals were fed a low-fat, high-carbohydrate diet for four weeks. At another time, the volunteers were fed a high-fat, low-carbohydrate diet for the same length of time.[16] Compared to the low-carbohydrate diet, the low-fat one led to a reduction in the size of the LDL particles (not a good thing). Also, adopting a low-carbohydrate diet has been found to induce a healthy increase in LDL particle size.[17]

Put all this together and what we have is evidence that low-carbohydrate diets have the potential to improve disease markers *across the board.*

Carbohydrate and Cardiovascular Disease

The logical conclusion to draw from this, of course, is that a diet rich in carbohydrate has the capacity to actually worsen disease markers. But that's not the only risk from eating such a diet: disruption in blood sugar has been shown to induce processes that encourage disease, and cardiovascular disease in particular.[18] Effects here include:

- Increased inflammation (a key underlying process in cardiovascular disease).

- Increased 'oxidative stress' (also known as 'free radical' damage) – another potential underlying process in many chronic diseases including cardiovascular disease.

- Protein glycation (the binding of glucose to proteins in the body, thereby damaging them).

- Increased coagulation (essentially making the blood 'stickier' and more likely to clot).

- Raised blood levels of triglycerides (a known risk factor for cardiovascular disease).

Overall, high GI or GL diets are associated with an increased risk of cardiovascular disease of the order of between 20 and 100 per cent.[18] A major review also concluded that there is compelling evidence to suggest that high GI or GL diets actually *cause* heart disease.[19]

Now, remember, for decades we've been enthusiastically encouraged to swap saturated fat for carbohydrate for the sake of the health of our heart. But, as we learned in Chapter 12 (A Matter of Fat), there is no good evidence that saturated fat causes heart disease. There is evidence, however, that certain carbohydrates that we've been encouraged to eat should be consumed with caution. So what does happen when individuals follow advice to cut back on saturated fat and eat more carbohydrate instead?

In one study, eating habits and risk of heart disease were assessed in more than 53,000 individuals over more than a decade.[20] The researchers found that substituting high GI carbohydrates for saturated fat was associated with a 33 per cent *increase* in risk of heart attack. Another study (this one a meta-analysis of 11 studies) found that swapping carbohydrate for saturated fat was associated with an enhanced risk of 'coronary events' such as heart attack.[21]

This evidence is epidemiological but, remember, it's underpinned by research finding that blood sugar-

GRAIN OF TRUTH

disruptive carbohydrates induce disease-causing processes in the body.

Taken as a whole, the research reveals that taking saturated fat out of the diet and putting carbohydrate in its place will, at best, do nothing to reduce the risk of heart disease. At worst, though, there's good reason to believe this basis of 'healthy' eating actually increases disease risk.

Just How Nutritious Are Grains Anyway?

One common concern about restricting starchy carbohydrates such as bread and breakfast cereals in our diet is that in so doing we will be missing out on essential nutrients. However, while it's often taken for granted that grains, particularly wholegrains, are packed full of nutrients, is this really the case?

One way to assess the nutritional value of a food is to compare the level of nutrients in it with its calorie content, the idea being that the best foods are those of the higher nutrient content but the lowest caloric load. This has led researchers to develop a concept known as the 'nutrient density score'.[22]

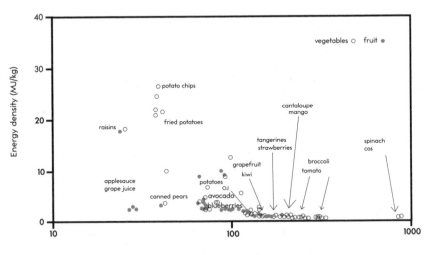

Figure 6: Relation between energy density and the naturally nutrient rich score for fruits and vegetables

ESCAPE THE DIET TRAP

Figure 6 summarizes the assessments for fruits and vegetables, generally regarded as nutritious foods. The healthiest foods are those that are positioned low (low-energy density) and to the right (high-nutrient levels) on the graph. Looking at the figure we can see that fresh fruits and vegetables, with the exception of the potato, generally rate very well indeed.

Now compare these results with those obtained for grains as seen in Figure 7. As you can see, generally speaking grain foods are higher in energy density and lower in terms of their nutritional offering. This includes wholegrain foods such as wholemeal bread.

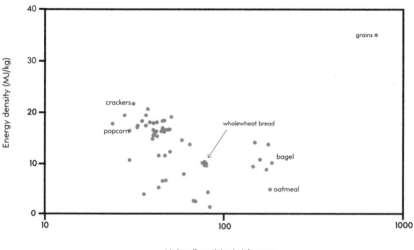

Figure 7: Relation between energy density and the naturally nutrient rich score for grains

In this figure, refined carbohydrates such as regular pasta, white bread and white rice are not labelled. However, bearing in mind that even wholegrains turn out not to be that nutritious, it doesn't look good for refined grains. The *un*-nutritious nature of grains is strongly suggested by the fact that many grain-based foods including bread and breakfast cereals are 'fortified' with additional nutrients. If they are inherently nutritious, why fortify them?

GRAIN OF TRUTH

It's also worth bearing in mind that some grains, notably wholewheat grains, contain substances called 'phytates' that block the absorption of nutrients such as calcium, magnesium, iron and zinc. So not only do many grains lack much in the way of nutrients, they can actually stop us getting nutritional value from them and the foods we eat with them.

The bottom line is that while many starchy carbohydrates are technically food, they are actually better described as *fodder*. You may be familiar with refined sugar being described as 'empty calories', a reference to the fact that it has the potential to fatten and offers very little in the way of nutritional value. I'd encourage you to think about grain-based foods including bread, rice and breakfast cereals in a similar way.

Where's My Fibre Going to Come From?

A common theme in messages we receive regarding the 'necessity' of grains in the diet is that they are rich in fibre – something that is claimed to be good for bowel health. The sort of fibre that is generally being referred to here is known as 'insoluble' fibre, more colloquially referred to as 'bran' or 'roughage'. This is said to provide bulk to our stools, and help prevent constipation and colon cancer.

Actually, insoluble fibre can be an irritant to the gut, and provoke symptoms such as bloating and discomfort. On the other hand, the other main form of fibre – 'soluble' fibre – tends to improve bowel symptoms such as constipation and abdominal discomfort.[23] Soluble fibre is found abundantly in natural foods such as fruit, vegetables, nuts and seeds.

The idea that insoluble fibre helps prevent colon cancer is not supported by the research either. For example, studies show that supplementing the diet with fibre does not reduce the risk of cancerous tumours or pre-cancerous lesions.[24-26]

The authors of a recent review concluded that '... there does not seem to be much use for fiber in colorectal diseases', adding that their desire was to 'emphasize that what we have all been made to believe about fiber needs a second look. We often choose to believe a lie, as a lie repeated often enough by enough people becomes accepted as the truth'.[27] I believe that last observation applies to the majority of received nutritional 'wisdom'.

Against the Grain

It's well recognized in medicine that foods can sometimes trigger unwanted reactions in the body. In their most extreme form, these reactions cause 'anaphylactic shock' that can be life-threatening. However, other types of reactions to food can occur, too, that, although not as obvious and less well recognized, can nonetheless have debilitating effects on health.

Food sensitivity issues – often referred to as 'food intolerance' – can be at the root of a range of health issues. While any foodstuff may do this, in practice grains are a common cause of problems. Grains contain proteins known as lectins that the human digestive tract finds difficult to digest. This job is not made any easier by the fact that grains also contain what are known as 'protease inhibitors' that impair protein digestion. The end result is that lectins can remain relatively intact in the gut.

The problem here is that lectins can be absorbed into the gut wall or through it into the bloodstream, and can be recognized as something 'foreign', rather like a bacterium or virus. The body's response to this is different from the one it would use to protect itself from an invading organism. This can cause problems in the gut (including discomfort and 'leakiness' in the gut wall that can further allow absorption into the body of potential toxins). The immune responses to food may 'overspill' to other parts of the body and cause one or more of a wide variety of symptoms including headaches, sinus congestion, asthma, eczema, rheumatoid arthritis and fatigue.

As I have said, grains are frequently at fault here and one grain that is particularly troublesome in this respect is *wheat* (found in, among other things, most forms of bread, breakfast cereals, biscuits, cakes, pastries, pasta and pizza). Wheat is particularly rich in a specific lectin known as 'wheat germ agglutinin'.

Wheat is also a source of *gluten* – another protein that the body can have difficulty dealing with. Some individuals have extreme sensitivity to gluten in the form of what is known as 'coeliac disease'. This causes 'flattening' of finger-like projections in the small bowel, hindering the absorption of food. It can cause digestive symptoms including pain, bloating and diarrhoea, as well as malnutrition.

Blood tests for gluten sensitivity exist, and it can also be diagnosed through biopsy of the small bowel. Positive tests pretty much assure that someone has a problem with gluten. However, negative tests do not rule out a problem with gluten. There is evidence that some individuals react to gluten even though they do not have coeliac disease.[28] Gluten is not just found in wheat but also in other grains, including oats, rye and barley.

Grain on the Brain

One other problem with certain grains is that they can be quite *addictive*. Gluten in the body can form what are called 'morphine-type peptides', or 'gluteomorphins', that attach to the same receptors in the brain that morphine binds to. In this way, gluten-containing grains, particularly wheat, can have slightly euphoric and therefore addictive potential for some people.

My experience in practice and also scientific data suggest that many grains (and in particular wheat) have the potential to do a lot of harm in the body. To summarize, grains:

1. Generally disrupt blood sugar levels in a way which predisposes to fatigue, mood problems, waking in the night, hunger and sweet cravings.

2. Tend to induce surges of sugar and insulin that predispose to issues such as weight gain, Type 2 diabetes and heart disease in the long term.

3. Are generally *un*-nutritious.

4. Contain phytates that impair the digestion of key nutrients.

5. Are rich in lectins and may also contain gluten that predispose to digestive issues and food sensitivity issues including arthritis, asthma and eczema.

6. Contain protease inhibitors that impair the digestion of proteins including lectins and gluten.

7. May be addictive (gluten-containing grains such as wheat).

With all this in mind, does it really make sense for grains to form the cornerstone of our diets, as our governments and health experts advise?

Does all this bad news mean we should eat no grain at all? Not necessarily. Some individuals seem to tolerate grain products reasonably well, but my experience is that such individuals are rare birds. My overwhelming experience in practice is that when individuals eat less of these foods (or none at all), they usually experience palpable benefits in terms of weight loss, general health and their sense of vitality.

WHERE'S MY ENERGY GOING TO COME FROM?

One concern regarding low-carbohydrate eating is that it will cause the body to run short on the sugar it 'needs' to fuel itself. First of all, a 'low-carb' diet does not mean 'no-carb'. Even if the diet was completely devoid of starchy carbohydrate and added sugar, some carbohydrate will still be available to the body in the form of, say, vegetables.

But let's imagine for a moment that someone were to eliminate every last molecule of carbohydrate from their diet and eat nothing but protein and fat. What would happen then? As we learned in Chapter 7, the body has the capacity to convert protein into

GRAIN OF TRUTH

glucose in a process known as 'gluconeogenesis'. It has been estimated that about 200 g of glucose can be generated this way each day, considerably more than enough to meet the body's requirement for carbohydrate.

It's a plain and simple fact that the body's absolute requirement of dietary carbohydrate is actually none at all.

This is, by the way, in stark contrast to fat and protein, as these supply what are known as 'essential fatty acids' and 'essential amino acids' respectively that can *only be supplied via the diet.*

The Bottom Line

- Insulin is the chief driver of fat accumulation in the body.

- The higher the blood sugar level rises, the more insulin is secreted in response.

- The extent to which a food destabilizes blood sugar levels is expressed as its 'glycaemic index' (GI).

- The overall impact of a food on blood sugar and insulin levels will depend not just on its GI, but on how much of that food is eaten. This overall effect is described as a food's 'glycaemic load' (GL).

- Many grain-based foods including wheat, bread, white rice, rice cakes and breakfast cereals generally have high GIs and GLs.

- High GI and GL diets are associated with an increased risk of insulin resistance, Type 2 diabetes and heart disease.

- When carbohydrate is restricted, the body can derive energy from ketones formed from fat.

- Ketosis is a natural response to low carbohydrate availability and poses no health risk to the body.

- In the short term, blood sugar instability (from eating foods of high GI or GL) can cause blood sugar levels to drop, which may provoke symptoms such as fatigue, hunger, food cravings, mood issues and waking in the night.

- Low-carbohydrate diets lead to improvements in markers of disease risk including insulin sensitivity, blood pressure and blood fat levels.

- Compared with fruits and vegetables, grains are quite *un*-nutritious foods.

- Grains contain 'phytates' that impair the absorption of nutrients.

- Grains, and in particular wheat, are a common cause of food intolerance and can be addictive.

- The absolute dietary requirement for carbohydrate is none at all.

Chapter 15

SWEET AND SOUR

Sugar is found naturally in the diet, for example in fruit. However, the modern-day diet is generally rich in added sugar, derived from sugar beet, sugar cane and, increasingly, corn. In this chapter we're going to assess the potential for added sugar to contribute to obesity and disease.

Those keen to avoid sugar may substitute artificial sweeteners in its place. Although sweet, these boast virtually no calories while promising better weight control. In this chapter we'll also be examining if this idea stands up to scrutiny.

What Is Sugar?

Table sugar, the form of sugar individuals generally spoon into their tea or coffee, or use when making, say, cakes and puddings, is comprised of *sucrose*. Sucrose is technically a 'disaccharide', a term used to describe sugars which are comprised of two individual sugar molecules joined together. Those two sugars, in the case of sucrose, are *glucose* and *fructose*. When sucrose it consumed it is digested down to its constituent sugars prior to absorption into the bloodstream.

The glucose in sucrose undoubtedly contributes to the glycaemic load of the diet, and the more sugar someone eats, the greater the rise in blood sugar levels. As we learned in the last chapter, spikes in blood sugar can induce processes such as inflammation and blood clotting that would be expected to increase the risk of heart disease. Also, higher levels of sugar will mean higher levels of insulin, which will predispose to insulin resistance, Type 2 diabetes and, of course, weight gain.

What About Fructose?

In contrast to glucose, fructose has traditionally enjoyed a healthy reputation, mainly on the basis that it does not raise blood sugar levels directly. Fructose is also the predominant sugar in some fruits – something which tends to bestow on it an image of healthiness.

In recent years, though, a steadily growing mountain of research has demonstrated that fructose, while it does not raise blood sugar levels directly, can nevertheless have toxic effects on the body. Interest here has been sparked, at least in part, by the fact that increasing amounts of the sweetening agent 'high fructose corn syrup' (HFCS) are making their way into the diet. HFCS is made cheaply by the chemical treatment of corn, and contains fructose and glucose in roughly equal measure.

HFCS started to be used in food production in meaningful quantities in the 1970s, but these days contributes substantially to our diets as an ingredient in foods such as breakfast cereals, cereal bars, biscuits, cakes, ready made desserts, sweetened yoghurts and soft drinks, as well as some more savoury foods including cooking sauces, condiments (e.g. ketchup) and crackers.

Whatever its source, once fructose is absorbed into the body it is transported directly to the liver. Fructose must be metabolized here, because the rest of the body does not have the metabolic machinery required to deal with it. Some fructose is converted into glucose, and therefore fructose can raise glucose levels in the bloodstream, albeit indirectly.

The other major fate of fructose is actually *fat* – at least some of the products of the metabolism of fructose can be turned into fat through the process known as *de novo* lipogenesis in the liver (discussed in Chapter 6). It seems that some of this fat can get 'stuck' in the liver itself, creating 'fatty liver'.[1] Fructose has been implicated, too, in the condition metabolic syndrome, characterized by abdominal obesity, that we discussed in Chapter 3 (Toxic Waist).[2]

The fat formed through the metabolism of fructose can make its way into the bloodstream as triglycerides. In one study, men fed a fructose-rich diet for four weeks saw very significant increases in their triglyceride levels.[2] Among other things, high triglycerides may hamper the action of leptin, which might lead to slower metabolism and increased hunger. In fact, fructose has been linked with leptin resistance.[3,4] Fructose has also been found to have the potential to promote insulin resistance.[5,6] Perhaps not surprisingly, reviews link fructose consumption obesity and Type 2 diabetes, as well as raised blood pressure.[7,8]

There is therefore good evidence that fructose has considerable capacity to harm health. A similar claim could, though, be made for any element of the diet (*anything* can harm health if we consume enough of it). In the studies in which fructose has been fed to animals or humans, relatively large doses have been used which may not reflect normal levels of intake. Do we have any idea how much fructose is *too much*?

How Much Is Too Much?

One review concluded that fructose at levels of 25–40 g per day appears to be safe.[9] Another concluded that the safe limit is most probably something under 90 g per day.[10] My tendency would be to shoot for more conservative intakes, on the basis of a study which found that just 40 g of fructose each day in the form of a sweetened beverage for three weeks induced unhealthy changes, including raised markers of inflammation, increased 'waist-to-hip' ratio (suggesting worsening abdominal obesity) and unfavourable changes in the size of LDL-cholesterol particles.[11]

The situation is further complicated by the fact that, as with most things, there is individual variation in our ability to handle

SWEET AND SOUR

fructose safely. It is possible that someone could consume 100 g or more in a day without ill effect, while someone else may suffer through the consumption of much smaller quantities.

With all this in mind, here are a few generalities that I believe hold true:

- Fructose may not raise blood sugar levels directly, but most certainly is not benign in terms of its effects on health.

- There is convincing and consistent evidence in animals and humans that fructose can induce problems such as insulin resistance, leptin resistance, high blood pressure and weight gain.

- Relatively small amounts of fructose in the diet are likely to be safe for the majority of people, particularly when found naturally in a relatively healthy food such as fruit. An apple, for instance, contains about 6 g of fructose, compared to about 20 g found in a can of cola.

Are Artificial Sweeteners a Better Bet?

Artificial sweeteners such as aspartame, sucralose and saccharin offer sweetness with few or no calories, and would seem the obvious choice over sugar for those seeking to lose weight. However, to know for sure if artificial sweeteners have weight-loss benefits they would need to be subjected to what are known as 'randomised controlled' trials. These trials, often used to assess pharmaceuticals, are generally regarded as the gold standard trials required for determining something's effectiveness. Bearing in mind how much faith we're asked to put in artificial sweeteners, one would imagine there's plenty of evidence to support them.

Curiously, however, not one single randomized controlled trial assessing the effects of artificial sweeteners on weight is to be found in the scientific literature.

One explanation for this is that such studies have not been done. Another is that such studies *have* been done, but have not

ESCAPE THE DIET TRAP

been *published*. The practice of publishing welcome results, but binning those that are unwelcome, leads to what is known as 'publication bias'. This practice can give a very skewed version of reality.

It's hard to gauge whether publication bias has taken place in this area, but there's a lot of money in artificial sweeteners and it seems unlikely that one or more manufacturer would not seek evidence to prove their presumed benefits as weight-loss aids.

Also, there is some evidence, albeit in animals, that suggests artificial sweeteners might actually *contribute to* obesity. In one study, rats were fed with either saccharin or sugar-sweetened yoghurt together with their normal diet.[12] Compared to those eating sugar-sweetened yoghurt, the rats eating saccharin-sweetened yoghurt consumed more calories and got fatter, too. The authors of this study concluded that '… using artificial sweeteners in rats resulted in increased caloric intake, increased body weight, and increased adiposity [fatness]', adding that 'These results suggest that consumption of products containing artificial sweeteners may lead to increased body weight and obesity by interfering with fundamental homeostatic, physiological processes.'

One potential explanation for this phenomenon relates to the ability of artificial sweeteners to stimulate the appetite, something we shall explore in Chapter 17 (Appetite for Change).

The limited (if any) benefits of artificial sweeteners should perhaps not come as too much of a surprise when we consider that they are extremely recent additions to the human diet. The chances that we have the biochemical and metabolic machinery necessary to deal with them effectively are therefore very low. The likelihood of them having benefits for health will also be low. Their potential for toxicity, on the other hand, would be expected to be high. This is something that we're going to be examining in more depth in Chapter 18 (Prime Fuel).

Another relatively recent addition to the human diet is milk. In the next chapter we're going to look at what place this foodstuff and other dairy products have in the diet.

The Bottom Line

- Glucose can contribute to the glycaemic load of the diet, raise blood sugar levels and increase the risk of obesity and chronic disease.

- Fructose, while it does not raise blood sugar levels directly, can predispose to weight gain and health issues through a variety of mechanisms.

- Limited quantities of fructose, especially when found naturally in food (such as fruit), are unlikely to prove hazardous to the body, but large amounts, particularly as a food additive, should be avoided.

- There is no good evidence that artificial sweeteners are better than sugar for controlling weight.

- Evidence in animals shows that artificial sweeteners can *cause* weight gain.

Chapter 16

SACRED COW

Milk and other dairy products represent staples in the 'standard Western diet', and their importance for growth and bone health is consistently impressed upon us. Yet for the vast majority of our time on this planet we drank no milk other than mother's milk early in life, and yet the record shows our ancestors had strong and healthy bones. Does it really make sense that we need milk *now*?

In this chapter we're going to look at the purported benefits of milk as well as other dairy products, and assess their effects on our bones, body weight and general health.

Boning Up

When dairy products are recommended, particular emphasis is placed on their 'essential' role in the growth and development of bones during childhood and adolescence. Calcium is found in dairy products, and it's also a component of bone. The obvious conclusion to draw is that dairy products are good for our bones. Except that there is little or no evidence to support this idea.

In one review, the great majority of studies found no evidence that calcium or dairy consumption impacted significantly on bone health in early life.[1] Of the remaining studies, any apparent benefit was revealed to be small. In another review, calcium supplementation in children and adolescents was found to have no effect on bone density in the hip or spine, and only marginal benefits for bone density in the arm.[2] An accompanying editorial highlighted the lack of evidence for the benefits not only of calcium but also of dairy products for bone health.[3]

Dairy products don't do much for the bones of the young, but do they have anything to offer older people? The consumption of dairy has been widely advocated as a key nutritional component in the combating of the bone-thinning disease known as 'osteoporosis'. Again, the evidence as a whole does not support this claim.

In one study of 72,000 women followed over an 18-year period, their consumption of milk and calcium appeared to have no bearing on risk of hip fracture.[4] Another review found that 12 out of 14 studies showed no relationship between milk consumption and bone health in women after the age of 50.[5] A recent meta-analysis found no evidence of reduced hip fracture risk from greater intakes of milk in either women or men.[6]

In another meta-analysis, researchers looked at the relationship between *calcium intake* specifically and hip fracture.[7] Again, higher calcium intakes were not linked with reduced risk of fracture. This study found that calcium supplementation (compared to placebo) actually *increased* risk of hip fracture by 64 per cent.

The research shows that dairy products, and the calcium they provide, have limited benefits for bone health, and might even be harmful in this regard.

Sensitive Issues

In Chapter 14 (Grain of Truth), we examined how grains, particularly wheat, pose hazards as a result of 'food intolerance'. My experience in practice is that dairy foods are a quite frequent factor in food sensitivity issues, too.

For instance, among children I find that dairy products are a common cause of ailments such as asthma, eczema, ear infections, glue ear, frequent colds and recurrent tonsillitis. In adults, some of the most common problems associated with dairy sensitivity include excessive catarrh, sinus and/or nasal congestion, asthma, eczema and irritable bowel syndrome.

A potential provoking factor here is the protein found in milk and other dairy products such as casein. Pasteurization is believed to make milk proteins particularly difficult to digest, and therefore more problematic. This idea is certainly consistent with my experience in practice: many individuals can tolerate raw dairy products, but react to those that have been pasteurized.

I find that yoghurt is much better tolerated than milk. This might have something to do with the fact that the bacteria deployed in the fermentation process that forms yoghurt partially digests milk proteins,[8,9] making them easier to digest and therefore less problematic. An added benefit of yoghurt is that it contains less lactose than milk, and is generally better tolerated by individuals who are lactose intolerant.

In addition to helping the digestibility of dairy products, studies suggest that the organisms found in 'live' and 'bio' yoghurts have the potential to help alleviate gut-related problems such as constipation, diarrhoea and irritable bowel syndrome.

What About Other Dairy Products?

In practice, pasteurized cheese and cream seem to have similar potential to cause food sensitivity issues as yoghurt. Butter, I find, is generally very well tolerated indeed, and this may have something to do with the fact that it is exceedingly low in both protein and lactose.

Another common finding is that individuals who react to cow's milk-based products, do not react as badly (and may not react at all) to milk and dairy products derived from other animals such as sheep and goats. It has been suggested that milk from these animals is, compared to cow's milk, more similar to human breast milk, thereby making it easier to digest and more appropriate for our consumption.

Dairy and Weight Control

Dairy products stimulate insulin secretion, and they appear to do this to an extent greater than is predicted by their impact on blood sugar levels.[10] In theory, the insulin-stimulating nature of dairy products may hinder weight control, seeing as this hormone is a key player in the deposition of fat in the body. It should be borne in mind, though, that dairy products such as yoghurt and cheese are rich in protein, which stimulates the secretion of glucagon, in turn counteracting some of the fat-forming effects of insulin (see Chapter XX).

Another factor that mitigates the fattening potential of dairy products relates to their calcium content. Consumption of calcium has been shown, paradoxically, to *lower* calcium levels within fat cells, and this accelerates the process of lipolysis (breakdown of fat).[11] There is considerable evidence linking higher intakes of calcium and dairy products with reduced body fatness.[12]

It has been suggested that not just calcium, but other chemical constituents in dairy products somehow assist fat loss. There is evidence that supplementing the diet with dairy products (yoghurt) can enhance fat loss, including abdominal fat.[13] In one of these studies,[14] the group supplementing with yoghurt saw their waist circumferences shrink by an average of about 4.0 cm, compared to a reduction of only about 0.5 cm in individuals supplementing with calcium alone.

While dairy products theoretically have fattening potential due to their influence on insulin, the evidence suggests their incorporation in the diet is unlikely to be a barrier to weight loss, and may even help here.

Dairy and the Primal Principle

Dairy products are relatively recent additions to the diet, and cannot therefore be described as 'primal' foods. However, for those who tolerate them, they do have something going for them from a nutritional perspective in that they are relatively rich in

ESCAPE THE DIET TRAP

protein and fat, and relatively low in carbohydrate. In this sense their 'macronutrient make-up' reflects one that we know tends to be the best for fat loss and disease markers.

Another important attribute of dairy products is a general tendency to sate the appetite quite effectively. The relatively protein- and fat-rich nature of dairy products such as full-fat yoghurt, cream and cheese probably has something to do with this. In the next chapter we're going to be looking at other factors important for controlling appetite that make healthy eating and the benefits that come with it a relative breeze.

The Bottom Line

- Milk and dairy product consumption appears to have little or no benefit with regard to bone health in children and adults.

- Dairy products can cause food sensitivity-related conditions including asthma, eczema and irritable bowel syndrome.

- Milk is generally the worst tolerated dairy product of all and butter the best. Yoghurt, cheese and cream fall somewhere in between.

- Goats' and sheep's products are generally better tolerated than cows' milk-based products.

- Yoghurt eating has been found to facilitate fat loss.

Chapter 17

APPETITE FOR CHANGE

Keeping hunger properly under control is a prerequisite for making any dietary regime enjoyable and sustainable. We've previously explored how protein and fat pack more appetite-sating punch than carbohydrate. In this chapter we're going to look at other important nutritional strategies for keeping hunger at bay and our eating habits on the straight and narrow.

Hunger Is the Enemy

For many people seeking to lose weight hunger is taken as a sure sign that they are in calorie deficit, and therefore *must* be losing weight. However, as we explored in Chapter 4 (The Burning Issue), in time going hungry can stifle the metabolism. Brief periods of conscious calorie restriction are not the problem, but prolonged periods of dietary constraint and hunger are.

Even in the shorter term, though, an uncontrolled appetite poses a serious hazard in that it can drive us to eat inherently fattening foods and eat too much of them when we do.

Imagine coming home ravenously hungry after being out all day. You need something quick and filling. What's it to be? A chicken salad or grilled lamb chops with steamed and buttered broccoli? Probably not. More likely the order of the day will look something like a plateful of pasta or a bowl of cereal. It's the same at lunch, in that feeling famished usually drives an intense desire for 'filling' foods – usually bread. Of course, the other side of this is that ensuring we approach meals in a not-too-hungry state can take the challenge out of making healthy choices.

Counterintuitive though this may sound, the less hungry you ensure you are, the more weight you're likely to lose.

I have witnessed countless individuals lose weight rapidly, enjoyably and sustainably using the approaches outlined in this book without any undue hunger at all in the long term. It's the absence of undue hunger that allows healthy choices to be made easily and enjoyably.

So, how hungry should you let yourself get before you eat a meal? Imagine a scale where 0 represents no hunger at all and 10 means you're ravenous. I recommend eating when hunger is about a 6 or a 7.

Here are the two fundamental keys to managing your appetite:

- Eating the right food.

- Eating it regularly enough.

Let's take each in turn ...

Eating the Right Food

We covered this earlier, but let's quickly recap the salient points.

In general terms, the most effective diet for sating the appetite is one that is rich in protein and fat, and relatively low in carbohydrate. One major advantage of such a diet is that it facilitates loss of fat, which can then be metabolized by the body – just like that hibernating bear I mentioned earlier. Because liberated fat represents food to the body, it helps sate the appetite. Protein has inherent appetite-sating properties, too.

The differing abilities of foods to satisfy the appetite helps to explain how it can be that many of us will find that a handful of nuts (rich in protein and fat) can tame an overeager appetite very effectively, while eating a bucket of carb-rich popcorn the size of our head will not really touch the sides.

DOES A PRIMAL DIET SATISFY?

In Chapter 11 (The Primal Principle) the idea was put forward that the best diet for us is one based on 'primal' foods, and we have seen support for this in the form of research regarding the impact of diet on weight and health. Could it be that primal eating hits the spot where appetite control is concerned, too.

In one study, men were asked to eat either a primal diet or a Mediterranean diet for a period of 12 weeks.[1] The primal diet emphasized lean meat, fish, fruit, vegetables, eggs and nuts. The Mediterranean diet was based on wholegrains, low-fat dairy products, vegetables, fruit, fish, vegetable oils and margarine. Both diets were *ad libitum*.

Those eating the Mediterranean diet ate an average of over 1,800 calories per day – that's what it took to satisfy them properly. On the other hand, the 'primal' eaters' were as satisfied, but with less food (under 1,400 calories).

It seems a primal diet really does have the capacity to satisfy and prevent overeating without hunger.

Eating Regularly Enough

One potential cause of the unbridled hunger that can lead to us making some poor food choices is simply going too long between fuelling stops. The 'danger time' for most people, I find, is between lunch and dinner. It's not uncommon for eight or more hours to elapse between these meals. This is just too long for most people. If we haven't eaten anything in between, by the time we sit down to dinner we can be far too famished to be satisfied by something truly healthy.

Some individuals can safely get away with skipping meals occasionally, in that they can delay or even miss entirely a meal without having their appetite run out of control. In fact, later in the book (Chapter 22) we're going to be looking at how skipping meals may enhance weight loss and help someone push through a weight plateau effectively and safely.

However, for most people, most of the time, I recommend not going from lunch to a lateish dinner without eating anything in between. As I've already mentioned, nuts represent a good snack. They are generally very effective for satisfying the appetite, and in relatively small amounts, too. And, remember, as we learned in Chapter 6, nuts are not a fattening food. More guidance about nut eating can be found in Chapter 18 (Prime Fuel).

The ability of nuts to sate the appetite effectively is, by the way, in contrast to the usual snack of choice – fruit. For most people, eating an apple, orange or half a bunch of grapes will leave them as hungry or even hungrier than they were to begin with.

Hungry for More?

Eating when very hungry is not a good idea, but eating in the absence of much of an appetite isn't either – gratuitous eating generally does nothing to speed fat loss. As suggested earlier in this chapter, the aim is to eat when hunger is about a 6 or 7 out of 10.

From time to time our particular situation can make it hard for us to avoid eating when we are not hungry. For example, we may feel it impolite not to eat when our spouse or a relative has, say, cooked us a special meal, or if we're sitting down in a restaurant with business colleagues or clients. *Occasional* excursions such as these shouldn't concern us, though.

However, if you quite often find yourself eating when you're not hungry or continuing to eat once you're full, I suggest taking remedial action.

For some of us, eating in the absence of hunger can appear to be due to 'emotional eating'. Here, eating can seemingly be triggered by 'negative' emotions such as anxiety and sadness. More about this, and how to manage it, can be found below under the heading Emotional Eating (below).

However, for some people eating does not appear to be emotional in the traditional sense. And my experience is that the problem here is often habitual and down to *conditioning*. Repeated eating and overeating of food in the absence of true hunger (often in childhood) can cause us to become somewhat deaf to the appetite signals our body gives us. Here are some strategies that can help:

1. Get in tune with your hunger signals

Spend just a few seconds, several times each day, asking yourself just how hungry you really are. Rate your hunger on a scale of 0–10. Doing this will help you get back in touch with the signals your body uses to tell you how genuinely hungry you are.

2. Avoid eating 'by the clock'

Some individuals get into the habit of 'eating by the clock', for example having lunch because 'it's lunchtime' whether they are hungry or not. If you are aware that you do this, resolve, wherever practical, to delay eating until you are genuinely hungry.

3. Avoid 'clearing your plate'

One potential driver of unnecessary eating is the belief that we need to finish everything on our plate. If you think this applies to you, start by making a conscious effort to leave some food, however small, on your plate at the end of the meal.

4. Use smaller crockery

A meal that's big enough truly to satisfy may still look insignificant or lost on a large plate or in a big bowl. Using crockery that is appropriate for smaller sized but properly satisfying meals can reduce the tendency to pile food unnecessarily high.

5. Avoid 'eating for later'

Some individuals eat with the aim of avoiding hunger before the next meal. However, this can encourage overeating when the time between meals is long (e.g. between lunch and dinner). Aim to eat enough at each meal to be comfortably full. Remember that it's fine to eat a healthy snack (e.g. nuts) to tide you over to the next meal should you get peckish.

Getting the Balance Right

In Chapter 8 (Hunger No More), we explored how blood sugar lows (hypoglycaemia) can trigger hunger, and an urge to scoff carbohydrate in particular. Foods of choice tend to be something sweet such as chocolate bars, biscuits, pastries, cakes or sugary soft drinks. Cutting back on carbs, and putting more emphasis on protein and fat in the diet, really helps to stabilize blood sugar levels, and therefore are key tactics for quelling carbohydrate cravings in time.

However, if the body has been used to getting ready fuel in the form of fast-releasing carbohydrate, it can take a while for it to adjust to the sudden scaling back of sugar and starch. The carb cravings that can result threaten to derail even the most committed of healthy eaters. Should this happen to you, help is at hand ...

Supplementary Benefits

Blood sugar balance is regulated by processes that depend on the supply of specific nutrients, probably the most important of which is the mineral *chromium*. Supplementing with this nutrient does seem to help stabilize blood sugar levels and, very importantly, can help to curb carb cravings in particular.

In one study, overweight women treated with 1,000 micrograms (mcg) of chromium per day saw their hunger (and food intake) fall significantly compared to women taking a placebo.[2] In another study, chromium supplementation was found to reduce carbohydrate cravings specifically.[3]

Some supplements offer a blend of nutrients designed to help stabilize blood sugar. In addition to chromium, these often include magnesium and B vitamins. Such a supplement, or even straight chromium, can be very useful during the initial stages of transition to a lower carbohydrate diet. Whether in combination with other nutrients or alone, I recommend 400–800 mcg of chromium daily, spread out over 2–3 doses during the day.

Glutamine Can Help with Food Cravings, Too

Sugar cravings are usually triggered when the brain is starved of fuel. The amino acid glutamine (not to be confused with glutamate – a constituent of MSG – see below) provides ready fuel for the brain, and in practice can extinguish carbohydrate cravings.

I suggest buying glutamine as a powder and dissolving 1 teaspoon (about 4 g) in about 500 ml of water. This should be sipped throughout the day, particularly between meals as food cravings are more likely to strike then, but also because glutamine is better absorbed on an empty stomach.

Using chromium-containing supplements and additional glutamine can be highly effective in curbing cravings. Such measures are usually only required for, say, 2–6 weeks, after which it is generally possible to gradually reduce and then stop without the return of troublesome food yearnings.

Emotional Eating

Some individuals have labelled themselves 'emotional eaters'. The idea here is that they can feel driven to eat foods as a result of 'negative' states such as stress, anxiety or sadness. In a moment,

I'm going to suggest two approaches that I find generally very effective for dissolving emotional eating effectively and quickly. Before that, though, let's explore whether *emotional* eating is always as emotional as it appears to be.

Take someone who is prone to blood sugar instability. Should their blood sugar level drop, their body will usually respond by secreting 'stress' hormones such as adrenaline, one effect of which is to increase anxiety. In addition to changes in mood, low blood sugar levels can trigger cravings for foods that replenish sugar quickly into the bloodstream such as chocolate, biscuits or bread. Bingeing on these foods may ensue. But here's the question: what caused the craving and subsequent bingeing – the person's emotions, or the drop in blood sugar level that triggered those emotions in the first place?

In my experience, many individuals who believe they have an 'emotional eating' problem have, at the risk of sounding dismissive, nothing of the sort. How do I know? Because I've seen time and time again that when an 'emotional eater' eats properly, and in particular stabilizes their blood sugar levels, their 'emotional eating' problem simply disappears. In many individuals, what appears to be an eating issue rooted in psychology is, in reality, *physiological* in nature.

This is not to say that emotional eating cannot happen – it most certainly can. For example, after repeated offering of sweet foods as a treat or pacifier in childhood it is undoubtedly possible for individuals to associate such foods with certain emotions. If that is genuinely the case with you, then the following information and advice should help.

To understand how best to approach this issue, it helps to appreciate that the mind has *conscious* and *unconscious* components. The conscious mind is what, among other things, allows you to think about problems and rationalize and work them out. While you've been reading this book, for instance, it's likely that your conscious mind will have been quite active.

Many emotional responses, however, are seated in the unconscious mind which, as the term suggests, controls unconscious thoughts and behaviour. Many emotional responses are seated here. An example is my spider phobia. I am afraid of spiders, even though I know that here in the UK they can't hurt me in any meaningful way. Nevertheless, in my unconscious mind I associate spiders with some form of threat, hence my response. The thing is, no amount of talking it through with a therapist or attempting to rationalize this in my own mind is likely to make much difference. Taking a conscious approach to an unconscious problem is a bit like attempting to fix a misfiring engine without first flipping the bonnet.

To resolve a genuine emotional eating issue it helps to 'flip the bonnet'. Here are a couple of strategies that tend to work well:

Hypnotherapy

It might conjure up images of swinging fob watches but, in a therapeutic setting, hypnosis is really nothing like this. A hypnotherapist's job is to induce a state in which the conscious mind is 'shut off' a bit. Technically, this is termed 'trance', but for many people it really is no more trancelike than the state we can be in when we drive down a motorway, only to realize we have no recollection of our journey over the last few miles, or the feeling of being lost in a good book or piece of music.

Once a highly and suggestible state is induced, the hypnotherapist can then 'instruct' the unconscious mind to respond more appropriately to the usual emotional triggers.

Emotional Freedom Technique (EFT)

Even the term 'emotional freedom technique' puts some people off, but bear with me for a moment. This form of therapy involves the tapping of specific points on the body while focusing on an emotional (or even physical) issue. It can also involve counting, humming and moving the eyes in a particular sequence. There's no doubt about it, EFT can look and sound weird. But I've witnessed its ability to help individuals make huge strides forward in overcoming issues such as emotional eating.

One of the best things about EFT is that it can be self-taught and self-administered. Practitioners have their place, but I'm a big believer in individuals taking as much control of their health as possible into their own hands. EFT can be a powerful tool here. Plus, it's not just good for emotional eating – it can be applied to all sorts of issues, both physical and mental.

CHOCOLATE – TAKE A TRIP TO THE DARK SIDE

For those of us who like to treat ourselves to something sweet and self-indulgent from time to time, my advice is to opt for dark chocolate (70 per cent cocoa solids or more). One reason for this is that cocoa is actually quite a nutritious substance in its own right, and particularly rich in plant chemicals known as 'polyphenols' that are linked with protection from heart disease. The darker the chocolate, the more cocoa it contains and, importantly, the less sugar. Less sugar means less potential for blood sugar disruption and the reduced risk of craving for unhealthy carbs this can provoke.

Another reason why dark chocolate is to be preferred over milk chocolate is that it is, gram for gram, more satisfying than milk chocolate,[4] which might have something to do with its higher protein, lower GI nature. There's a tendency for people to eat less of it as a result.

One other reason for choosing dark chocolate over other varieties is that, well, it's just not *that* nice. In the mouth, dark chocolate lacks the texture and sweetness of milk chocolate, and it's not nearly as moreish as a result. A couple of squares of dark chocolate can be an indulgent way of rounding off an evening meal without engendering feelings of remorse or guilt.

The Appetite Disrupters

Eating the right foods regularly enough to keep the appetite under control will go a long way to making sure healthy eating is easy and enjoyable. However, it can nonetheless help to be aware that certain substances can divert us. Specific food additives have the capacity to stimulate the appetite and encourage us to consume calories that are surplus to requirements. The main known offenders here are monosodium glutamate (MSG) and artificial sweeteners.

MSG

Monosodium glutamate is a food ingredient used to enhance flavour and palatability. Although it's found in a wide range of processed food, for some time there have been lingering concerns about MSG's effects on health and weight.

MSG is known to have the capacity to stimulate the appetite, which is at least one reason it is used to lace many fast and processed foods. In animals, MSG does not just cause them to eat more,[5] but also stimulates insulin secretion.[6] There is the potential, therefore, that insulin secretion will lead to low blood sugar (hypoglycaemia) some time later, a side effect of which can be ravenous hunger. This might help to explain how it is possible to eat a big Chinese meal (MSG is commonly used in Asian cooking) only to find oneself absolutely famished just a couple of hours later.

Evidence links higher MSG intakes with enhanced risk of overweight or obesity.[7,8] In both of these studies the association remained even when factors such as overall food intake and activity levels were accounted for. In other words, it appears that MSG might cause weight gain in ways that are distinct from the appetite-stimulating effects it has.

One mechanism that may explain this is MSG's capacity to disrupt the functioning of the hypothalamus in the brain, which might induce leptin resistance. Also, animal experiments show that MSG has the capacity to suppress lipolysis (fat breakdown).[9]

One way to minimize your exposure to glutamate is to scrutinize labels for sources of this substance. Such sources to look out for include MSG (obviously), hydrolysed vegetable protein (HVP), hydrolysed plant protein, textured protein, autolysed plant protein, yeast extract, autolysed yeast and vegetable protein extract.

Of course, if you find you need to inspect the ingredients label of a particular food, you probably haven't got the best food in your hand in the first place. If your diet is primarily made up of natural, unprocessed foods like meat, fish, eggs, fruit, vegetables and nuts, then there's not much opportunity for MSG to sneak in. While you're steering clear of processed foods, give a wide berth to fast food, too, as this is another major source of MSG in the diet.

Artificial Sweeteners

Artificial sweeteners come with a weight-loss promise, though in Chapter 15 (Sweet and Sour) we discovered that there is actually no good evidence for this at all. In that chapter I also touched on research which finds that animals fed artificially sweetened foods actually grew fatter than those eating sugar-sweetened food.

One explanation for this is that artificial sweeteners can stimulate the appetite through effects on the brain. In one study, women were given a solution containing either the artificial sweetener sucralose or sucrose (table sugar).[10] The women were unable to distinguish the source of the sweetness on the basis of taste. However, it seems their brain knew the difference: sugar activated 'pleasure centres' in the brain more than sucralose. It seems an artificial sweetener may simply not give the level of pleasure and satisfaction derived from sugar. This, in theory, could lead individuals to seek satisfaction from other foods (i.e. to eat more).

Some evidence shows that artificial sweeteners have the ability to stimulate the appetite. For example, one study revealed that women given aspartame-sweetened lemonade were found to consume considerably more calories overall compared to those drinking regular (sugary) lemonade.[11] In another study, researchers found that subjects who had eaten yoghurt sweetened with saccharin were inclined to eat more than those who had eaten yoghurt sweetened with sugar.[12] There is further evidence which suggests that aspartame has the capacity to stimulate the appetite when ingested in chewing gum.[13] Sugar-sweetened foods are far from ideal, but it does seem that artificially sweetened ones are simply not a good alternative.

What about more natural sweeteners? Some sweeteners like stevia and xylitol are marketed as healthier alternatives to artificial sweeteners such as aspartame and sucralose. They may indeed be safer, but here's my problem with them: they're *sweet*. I know that's the whole point, but the issue here is that their consumption further accustoms us to sweet, potentially quite addictive, tastes. I believe it's better for individuals to eschew any attachment to sweetness in the long term. Most individuals find that within a couple of weeks of following the advice outlined in this book they've lost any sweet tooth they ever felt they had.

Speed-Eating Can Lead to Overeating

You probably won't find the fact that the hungrier we are the quicker we tend to eat much of a revelation. However, the important thing is that the faster we eat, the *more* we may end up eating before the brain tells us that we've had enough. In one study, men who ate quickly were found to be almost twice as likely to be overweight compared to those taking more time over their food.[14]

The question is, could slowing down and chewing food more thoroughly help to prevent overeating? In one study, 30 women were asked to eat a pasta-based meal under two distinct conditions.[15] At one sitting, they were asked to take small bites and chew each one 15–20 times. At another sitting, they were asked to eat as quickly as possible. In this scenario, the women consumed about 70 calories more, and felt less satisfied immediately after the meal and also an hour later.

Other evidence for the potential importance of slowing our eating has come in the form of a study in which chocolate custard was fed to volunteers under a number of different conditions.[16] On one occasion, individuals were instructed to consume the custard by taking relatively small mouthfuls. At another time, they were asked to take mouthfuls three times as large. In both of these scenarios, but on different occasions, test subjects were also asked to process the food in their mouths quickly (3 seconds before swallowing) and slowly (9 seconds per mouthful). In all test settings, individuals were instructed to eat as much as they wanted and to stop when they had had enough.

One notable finding from this study was that individuals ate less when they took small mouthfuls compared to when they took larger ones. Average intake was about 100 fewer calories (about a 23 per cent calorie reduction). Also, though, the longer the food stayed in the mouth, the less was actually eaten.

Taking small mouthfuls and chewing them thoroughly may lead to a natural and unconscious reduction in the amount of food consumed during a meal.

Here Comes the 'Chew-Chew' – Tips for Slower Eating

1. Avoid getting too hungry before meals

This is the most important thing of all – it's very difficult to eat in a controlled fashion and savour food if you're ravenous. Eat the right foods regularly enough to ensure your appetite never runs riot.

2. Put less on your fork or spoon

Be conscious of how much food you're putting into your mouth. If you're stacking your fork or piling your spoon high with food, you might want to reconsider this. Make a conscious effort to keep each mouthful small and manageable.

3. Chew thoroughly

Thorough chewing not only aids digestion, but also slows down the eating process. Make a conscious effort to chew each mouthful of food about 20 times before swallowing. While you are chewing, put your cutlery down and don't pick it up again until you've fully chewed and swallowed the last mouthful. At the very least, even if you are going to keep hold of your cutlery, do not reload your fork or spoon until the previous mouthful has been thoroughly chewed and swallowed.

4. Savour food

Have you ever eaten a meal or snack and hardly tasted it? If so, the chances are that rapid, distracted eating was a factor. It's not always possible to take time over eating, but when the occasion allows, savour whatever it is you are eating and *enjoy* it.

EASY PICKINGS

In this chapter the importance of not getting too hungry before eating has been emphasized. This same approach should also be applied to food shopping. Going around the supermarket or convenience store in a ravenous state is asking for trouble. Having a satisfied stomach makes putting exclusively healthy foods in your basket or trolley far easier. Some people find online shopping a good tactic, too, in that it protects against visual and smell-related cues that can make it harder to resist tempting but frankly unhealthy foods such as bread, doughnuts and pastries.

The Bottom Line

• Keeping the appetite under control is key to healthy eating and sustainable weight loss.

- A satisfying diet will generally be one that is relatively rich in protein and fat and low in carbohydrate.

- Regular meals, and possibly snacks, can be important for regulating appetite and food intake.

- Episodes of low blood sugar (hypoglycaemia) can stimulate hunger and, in particular, cravings for carbohydrate.

- Chromium and other nutrients including magnesium and certain B vitamins can help stabilize blood sugar levels and combat food cravings.

- Glutamine provides ready fuel for the brain and can be effective in combating food cravings, too.

- MSG can stimulate the appetite and should be avoided.

- Similarly, artificial sweeteners can disrupt the appetite and predispose to weight gain.

- Eating slowly, chewing thoroughly and savouring food can all help prevent overeating.

- Avoid shopping for food when hungry.

ESCAPE THE DIET TRAP

Chapter 18

PRIME FUEL

The earlier chapters in this book exposed a myriad of reasons why conventional dieting, and low-fat, calorie-restricted diets in particular, so often fail to bring lasting weight loss. We went on to see how diets more limited in carbohydrate and richer in protein and fat than is traditionally advised are the most effective for weight control. An added boon is the fact that this way of eating for weight loss does not depend on conscious restriction of calories or portion control (so no hunger in the long term).

The middle part of this book extended our knowledge of nutrition beyond its impact on weight, and into health. We explored the relationship between major food types including fats, sugars, grains and dairy products and wellbeing and risk of diseases such as Type 2 diabetes and heart disease. The research here was put in the context of the idea that the best diet for us will be one which mirrors the diet on which we evolved. It turns out that the common sense of 'primal' eating is matched by the scientific evidence.

This chapter brings all this information together, and rates individual foods on the basis of what we know about their effects on weight and health. Other important information not covered previously will also be used to provide practical guidance on which foods we should emphasize in the diet and which are best left alone. Before we go into detail, let's remind ourselves of what we've learned so far.

A Quick Recap

The best diet for us will be one made up of natural, unprocessed foods, particularly those that reflect our 'primal' past. Emphasis should be placed on consuming more fat than we're generally urged to. Fats found naturally in food are neither fattening nor harmful to health. Some fats, most notably omega-3, are positively beneficial to health and may even assist weight loss. Industrially processed fats should be avoided.

Protein should be given some priority, too. Protein is the macronutrient that is most sating, and also has hormonal effects that counteract the fat-storage effects of insulin. Protein-rich diets might possibly assist weight loss through some 'metabolic advantage' too. Common concerns around protein with regard to heart, kidney and bone health are unfounded.

Carbohydrate is generally over-emphasized and over-consumed. The carbohydrate foods most important to limit are those that contain added sugar and/or are starchy (remember, starch *is* sugar). These are generally disruptive to blood sugar and insulin levels in a way that predisposes to weight gain, Type 2 diabetes and heart disease.

Artificial additives should be avoided, especially MSG and artificial sweeteners, as evidence suggests these have the capacity to promote weight gain.

Eating a diet made up of natural, unprocessed foods will also help meet our requirements for 'micronutrients' (vitamins and minerals), 'phytochemicals' (plant-derived substances which have health-promoting and disease-preventative properties) and soluble fibre.

Let's see how specific foods measure up according to these criteria. Any positive or negative features of each foodstuff will be highlighted. The food will also be given an overall rating as to whether it is to be eaten freely, in moderation or not at all (except, perhaps, in very small amounts). These ratings are summarized in Table 8 at the end of this chapter.

WHAT DOES 'MODERATION' MEAN?

Some of the foods here are recommended 'in moderation'. But what does *moderation* mean? It means, in essence, that wherever possible you should opt for foods that can be eaten in 'unlimited quantities'. However, when it becomes difficult to eat foods exclusively from this category, or you just fancy something else, then it's OK to eat something from the 'in moderation' list. This might be some bacon at breakfast, for instance, or a hunk of cheese as part of a late afternoon snack or mini-meal.

In the early stages of adjusting your diet, I recommend having a modest portion of an 'in moderation' food no more than once a day. However, once you are close to or have achieved your health goals, you can relax this. Even when you do, though, it is important to ensure that the bulk (about 80 per cent) of your diet is made up of 'eat freely' foods.

Meat

Meat is a satisfying, high-protein, low-carbohydrate food and ideal for individuals wanting to lose fat. The saturated fat in meat has not been shown to be hazardous to health and may even have some benefits. We also learned that fresh meat consumption is not linked with chronic diseases such as heart disease and Type 2 diabetes (see Chapter 12). It's also worth bearing in mind that about half the fat in meats such as lamb and beef is *monounsaturated* (heart-healthy) in nature.

Meat is rich in minerals, too, including iron (important for energy production and an essential component of the haemoglobin in red blood cells, which carries oxygen around the body), and zinc (which plays an important role in, among other things, immune function, wound healing, brain function and fertility). As far as vitamins are concerned, meat offers a rich complement of B vitamins, including B1 (thiamin), B2 (riboflavin), B3 (niacin), B6 and B12. These nutrients have a wide range of roles in the body and assist both in the generation of energy and in the balanced working of the brain.

Another of meat's nutritional benefits comes in the form of carnitine, a substance that helps the conversion of fat into energy in the body's cells. Meat is also rich in the amino acid leucine, which is important for muscle maintenance and growth, and which studies show helps prevent muscle loss during weight reduction.[1]

Meat Quality

Many commercially reared animals are intensively farmed, and are often exposed to drugs and chemicals that taint their meat. One of the worst in this respect is chicken. While poultry is generally regarded as healthier than 'red' meats such as beef and lamb, I have my doubts about this. Most chickens bred for food are kept in miserable conditions and loaded with growth-promoting antibiotics during their brief lives.

Chicken is one meat almost certainly worth eating in its organic, free-range form. The same is also true of pork, which is another usually intensively reared meat. An alternative to going organic is to choose wild game meats such as venison, pigeon, partridge, pheasant, wild boar, rabbit and duck.

There is evidence that the type of feed animals eat during their lives affects the nutritional profile of the meat they produce. Animals such as cows and sheep are herbivores that are adapted to eating grass. Yet in the intensive rearing of animals, grass is often substituted with grain (e.g. processed corn) and soya. Compared to animals fed these artificial foods, grass-fed ones contain higher levels of omega-3 fats.[2] When possible, and when your pocket allows, choosing grass-fed over grain-fed beef is a healthier bet all round.

The processing of meat is another potential concern. There is a world of difference between an unadulterated organic, free-range chicken and a chicken nugget. The latter is likely to contain poor-quality meat and numerous additives. Also, processed meats such as bacon, sausage and salami generally contain preservative chemicals such as sodium nitrite, which has links with stomach cancer[3] and brain tumours.[4]

DOES RED MEAT CAUSE COLON CANCER?

One form of cancer that is often said to be related to meat eating, particularly red meat, is colon cancer. It should be borne in mind that the supposedly 'incriminating' evidence here is epidemiological in nature (i.e. it cannot show that red meat *causes* colon cancer). Also, not all of the evidence is as you might expect.

For example, one review found that 31 of 44 epidemiological studies showed no apparent association between eating red meat and the risk of colon cancer.[5] This review highlighted the fact that links between meat consumption and colon cancer are much stronger for processed meat than for fresh red meat. This observation is backed by other evidence.[6]

It's difficult to draw conclusions from this sort of epidemiological data, but chemicals used to preserve meat such as sodium nitrite are believed to have some cancer-causing potential. If we're going to eat meat, I think this should come predominantly in the form of fresh meat from animals reared as naturally as possible, rather than processed meats such as sausages, ham, bacon and salami.

Summary

- Meat can be eaten freely (organic and/or naturally reared meat is preferred).

- Processed meats should be eaten in moderation.

ETHICS AND THE ENVIRONMENT

Some people have ethical concerns regarding the eating of animals and perhaps even animal-derived foodstuffs such as eggs and dairy products. I understand these concerns, but I don't share them. I do, however, respect people's right to choose to eat (or not eat) whatever they like. However, I think it's important also to distinguish between *ethical* concerns and *health* concerns. Overall, the evidence strongly supports the idea that an omnivorous diet is not only *not* harmful to health, it is positively health-giving. I personally have concerns about aspects of animal welfare, and support humane treatment of animals during rearing and slaughter.

Environmental concerns are valid, too, I think. Yet, while the rearing of animals for human consumption is often portrayed as utterly wasteful and destructive, there are quite powerful arguments for livestock farming, in that animals are an important part of our ecosystem. It's beyond the scope of a nutrition book to explore this issue in depth, but the issues are explored in Simon Fairlie's book *Meat: A Benign Extravagance* (2010).

Grain- and cereal-based agriculture should not be let off the hook either, in that it is generally hugely destructive to the environment and soil and disrupts ecosystems too. For those wishing to learn more about some of the salient points I recommend Lierre Keith's *The Vegetarian Myth* (2009).

Fish and Seafood

Fish and seafood (such as prawns, crab and mussels) are both rich in protein and low in carbohydrate. Like meat, they are good foods for individuals seeking to maintain a healthy weight. Fish and seafood are also generally good sources of zinc and iodine (important for the proper functioning of the thyroid gland). One other potential constituent of seafood and fish is vitamin D, which, among other things, plays a part in bone and muscle health. Mounting evidence also links higher levels of vitamin D with a reduced risk of chronic diseases, including cancer and cardiovascular disease.

Some forms of fish, notably salmon, mackerel, trout, sardines and herring, are rich in omega-3 fats. However, some questions have been raised about potential contaminants such as mercury (found, for example, in tuna, marlin and swordfish), which is toxic to the nervous system. Fish, particularly farmed, may be contaminated by substances such as dioxins and polychlorinated biphenyls (PCBs), which are believed to have cancer-promoting properties. When the overall impact of fish eating on health was assessed,[7] the conclusion was that it does more good than harm.

Another potential cause for concern is the depleted fish stocks in our seas. As a result, fish farming is now on the increase to meet demand. Fish farming exposes fish to chemicals (such as antibiotics and colourings) that are not encountered in the wild, and this is bad news from an ecological perspective.

In an ideal world, fish is best consumed in its wild rather than farmed form. However, fresh fish is generally expensive, and we need to be mindful of the rapidly depleting fish stocks in our seas. For a guide to the best fish to eat in terms of sustainability and from an ecological point of view, see www.fishonline.org.

Canned fish, though perhaps nutritionally not as good as fresh, can offer a more cost-effective way of consuming fish. Tinned tuna is popular, though much of the omega-3 fat this fish naturally contains is removed prior to canning. Tuna is also one of the fish that tends to be contaminated with mercury (see above). Better types of tinned fish to eat include salmon, mackerel and sardines: these are richer in omega-3 fatty acids and tend not to be contaminated with mercury.

Summary

- Fresh fish and seafood can be eaten freely.

- Tuna, marlin and swordfish should be eaten in moderation.

- Tinned fish other than tuna can be eaten freely.

CHINA CRISIS

2005 saw the publication of a book entitled *The China Study* by researcher T. Colin Campbell. It was based on epidemiological research conducted in China (referred to in the book as 'the China Study') which Campbell claims provided a powerful argument for avoiding cholesterol and animal protein. The book also refers to laboratory work in which giving the milk protein *casein* to animals increased the risk of liver cancer. *The China Study* and the research on which it is based are commonly cited as evidence for the health-giving benefits of vegetarian and vegan eating.

In reality, *The China Study* is actually peppered with half-truths and misinformation.

For example, while casein was found to induce liver cancer in animal studies, the doses used in the experiments were massive compared to the doses humans might consume. An important omission is the fact that another protein in milk – whey – has been found to *reduce* risk of liver cancer in animals. Also, there is some doubt about how relevant this animal research is to human health.

Many of the book's conclusions are drawn from the China Study itself, which was epidemiological in nature. In this respect, however voluminous the data, they are of no use for discerning cause and effect. Taking the data at face value for a moment, though, *The China Study* did not reveal significant associations between animal protein and cancer, heart disease or overall risk of death. None of this, of course, supports Campbell's contention that animal protein should be eliminated from the diet.

One of Campbell's objections to animal protein is that it is associated with increased blood cholesterol levels, which, he claims, are associated with cancer. This observation would perhaps be strengthened by evidence of a link between protein and cancer, but the China Study yielded no such evidence. And neither did it find any links between cholesterol-rich food (such as meat and eggs) and cancer.

If you have an appetite for lengthy and thorough critiques of the China Study, I recommend the work of bloggers Denise Minger and Chris Masterjohn (see Resources section at the back of the book).

Eggs

Eggs, like meat, fish and seafood, are rich in protein and low in carbohydrate. This makes them a good food for individuals seeking to lose fat and/or build muscle. Along with red meat, eggs have generally been caught up in the anti-fat hysteria of the last few decades. However, we now know that such concerns are unfounded. Besides, the most plentiful type of fat to be found in eggs is actually monounsaturated (heart-healthy) in variety. These facts help explain why, as we saw in Chapter 12 (A Matter of Fat), eggs do not have strong links with heart disease.

In addition to monounsaturated fat, other nutrients supplied by eggs include B vitamins (especially vitamins B2 and B12), vitamin A and vitamin D.

Summary

- Eggs can be eaten freely.

Fruit

Fruits are generally nutritious foods offering, for example, relatively high levels of micronutrients (including vitamin C) as well as soluble fibre. Fruit is also rich in phytochemicals, including hesperidin (citrus fruits) and flavonols (apples). Both these phytochemicals are linked with a reduced risk of heart disease. Strawberries and other berries are rich in ellagic acid, which appears to have cancer-preventative properties.

One potential problem with fruit, though, is the fact that it is generally very rich in sugar, sometimes in the form of fructose (see Chapter 15). To my mind, there is no real comparison between eating an apple and eating a doughnut. Nonetheless, the high-sugar content of many fruits means they are not necessarily something to emphasize in the diet if fat loss and optimum health are our goals. This is particularly the case for individuals known not to tolerate carbohydrate well, such as diabetics and those who suffer from insulin resistance, metabolic syndrome or Type 2 diabetes.

Probably the best fruits are berries, as these are relatively low in sugar and also offer a great deal in terms of nutrient content. Avocado pears are another good choice, chiefly because they are relatively low in sugar and protein- and fat-packed compared to other fruits. Fruits such as apples, pears, peaches, nectarines, plums and citrus fruits should be eaten in moderation. Certain tropical fruits, including bananas, mangoes and pineapples, are very sugar-rich and are best eaten in very limited quantities until weight and health goals are met. Dried fruit is intensely sugary, and should be avoided except in small quantities.

Summary

- Berries and avocado can be eaten freely.

- Tropical fruits such as bananas, mangoes and pineapples should be eaten in small quantities only.

- All other fresh fruits can be eaten in moderation.

- Dried fruit should be eaten in small quantities only.

FRUIT, VEGETABLES AND AGROCHEMICALS

While fruit and vegetables should assume a generally prominent place in our diet, there is always the chance that they will come to our table laced with unwanted chemicals. A lot of fresh produce is quite liberally treated with agrochemicals such as pesticides and fungicides, designed to keep it free from attack by insects and moulds.

In 2011, the Environmental Working Group (EWG) in the US published a list of the most and the least pesticide-contaminated fruits and vegetables. Most contaminated produce (in order of decreasing contamination) included apples, celery, strawberries, peaches, spinach, nectarines, grapes, red peppers, potatoes, blueberries, lettuce and kale. The chemicals that lace these food are designed to kill things, and common sense dictates that the fewer of these chemicals we consume, the better. With this in mind, organic fruit and vegetables make better options. Otherwise, very thorough washing of fresh produce will at least help to reduce the effect that pesticides may have on our health. The EWG found that some of the least contaminated fruit and vegetables included onions, avocado, asparagus, kiwi fruit, cabbage, sweet potatoes and mushrooms.

Vegetables

Vegetables that grow above the ground, such as broccoli, cabbage, cauliflower and kale, are low in carbohydrate and generally highly nutritious (rich in, for example, folate, vitamin C, phytochemicals and soluble fibre), and are recommended foods.

Vegetables that grow below the ground, however, such as carrots, parsnips, swedes and sweet potatoes, are richer in carbohydrate and should be eaten in moderation. Squashes and pumpkins are also relatively carb-rich, and are not to be emphasized in the diets of those actively seeking to lose weight.

White potatoes should be avoided except in relatively small amounts (e.g. a couple of roast potatoes or a small number of new potatoes as part of a meal). See Miss Mash? (below) for alternatives.

Onions contain moderate amounts of carbohydrate, but tend not to be eaten in quantities likely to pose problems. Mushrooms are very low in carbohydrate and relatively rich in vitamin D and can be eaten in unlimited quantities.

MISS MASH?

Some meals, for example sausages or shepherd's pie, can somehow seem incomplete without mashed potato. Mashed potato, particularly if piled high, tends to cause considerable blood sugar and insulin disruption, and is therefore far from ideal for those seeking to shed fat. A good alternative, though, is mashed *cauliflower*. Steam or boil the cauliflower until done and then mash with butter, salt and pepper (and perhaps some cream). You could also replace ordinary potatoes with sweet potatoes; these are more nutritious and generally less disruptive to blood sugar levels.

Summary

- Green and leafy vegetables can be eaten freely, as can onions.

- Squashes, pumpkins, sweet potatoes, beetroots, carrots, swedes and parsnips should be eaten in moderation.

- White potato should be avoided except in very limited quantities.

THE COST OF LIVING

There's no doubt that eating the sort of diet recommended here tends to hit our wallets and purses more than the carbohydrate-dense and more processed diet that is the norm for many of us. Spending less than a pound on a whole loaf of bread can look like substantially better value than forking out several times that amount on a piece of grass-fed beef.

Some of this apparent additional cost can be offset by choosing, say, cheaper cuts of meat that are appropriately cooked to render them tender (e.g. slow-cooked stews and casseroles). Also, it's important to remember that when people shift the direction of their diet in a lower-carb/more primal direction, they usually automatically eat *less* (sometimes a *lot* less) because they are simply less hungry. There are obvious financial savings to be had here, of course.

Another area in which individuals may save is eating out. Many people who improve their diet feel compelled to prepare more food for themselves, and end up eating out less as a result. It can be nice to eat out, but it can be even nicer (not to mention more economical) to prepare and share a meal in the more relaxed atmosphere of one's own home.

One other thing worth bearing in mind is that broadly following the dietary recommendations here almost always leads to a stepwise improvement in individuals' energy levels, vitality and general health. Risk of ill health and chronic disease will be much lower, too, saving time and healthcare costs. In essence, eating properly allows people to lead healthier, happier and more abundant lives. Many people will reason that this is worth paying more for in terms of their food bills.

Beans and Lentils

Beans and lentils are collectively referred to as pulses, or 'legumes' (a class of foods that also includes peas and peanuts). Legumes are a relatively recent addition to the human diet (about 10,000 years ago), and have some capacity to trigger unwanted food-sensitivity reactions. Like grains, they are relatively rich in proteins called lectins that can be toxic to the body. Legumes also contain 'enzyme inhibitors' that impair the digestion of food[8] and can increase the risk of food sensitivity as well as reduce food's nutritional value. On the plus side, there is evidence that the lectins and enzyme inhibitors found in legumes can be at least partially deactivated by thorough soaking and cooking (see below).

The inherent problems legumes pose need to be weighed against the fact that beans and lentils are at least generally eaten in their 'whole' and quite unprocessed form, in stark contrast to the refined, nutrient-stripped forms of grain that are commonplace in the diet. Also, legumes generally have low GIs and GLs compared to grains, which is generally a good thing.

I'm not a particularly enthusiastic advocate of legumes, but I believe they can be included in moderation in the diet. If they're not eaten, nothing is lost, though.

PREPARING PULSES

The lectins and digestion inhibitors found in pulses can be deactivated, to a large degree, by appropriate preparation and cooking. As far as preparation is concerned, soaking is the key. If cooked from their dried state, they should first be soaked for several hours (generally 4–12 hours). The soaking water should then be discarded, and the beans should be rinsed before cooking in unsalted water (salt tends to toughen their skins).

An alternative to this lengthy preparation time is to buy canned pulses, though these should be rinsed thoroughly to remove as much added salt and sugar as possible.

Thorough cooking of legumes will not just help to nullify lectins and digestion inhibitors, but can also reduce the levels of certain starches in beans that can ferment in the gut and cause wind.[9] Lectin levels can be reduced and the general digestibility of beans improved through sprouting (germinating beans prior to consumption).

Summary

- Legumes should be consumed in moderation only.

Soya

Soya beans are perhaps the most widely consumed beans of all. Actually, the bean itself is rarely eaten, but food products prepared from components of the bean are. For example, the oil derived from soya beans finds its way into many processed foods. Also, the protein-rich part of the bean can be used as the basis for a wide range of foods including tofu, soya milk, tempeh and miso.

Despite its widespread use in the diet, soya is actually a relatively new food – soya was probably first cultivated no more than 3,000 years ago. Like other legumes, soya beans contain substances that can impair digestion. Although these toxic compounds can be deactivated or removed during the processing of soya beans, at least some of them are likely to remain in the finished product, which can have repercussions for health.

Soya beans also contain high amounts of phytates that impair the absorption of minerals including calcium, magnesium, iron and zinc. Cooking, unfortunately, does not destroy phytates, though levels can be reduced (but not necessarily eliminated) by fermentation to make foods such as tempeh and miso.

The processing of soya generally involves converting the soya beans into something known as soy protein isolate (SPI). Production of SPI takes place in factories where a slurry of soya beans is treated with acid and alkali to precipitate out the protein. During this process the product can become tainted with the metal aluminium (believed to be toxic to the brain).

The resultant protein-rich curd is spray-dried at a high temperature to produce a powder. SPI may then be heated and extruded under pressure to make a foodstuff known as 'textured vegetable protein' (TVP). SPI and TVP will often have MSG added to them to impart a 'meaty' flavour. Once flavoured, SPI can be shaped into a wide range of foods including meat-substitute products such as vegetarian burgers, sausages and mince.

Certain toxins found in soya, including digestion inhibitors, are known to remain in SPI.[10] Animal research suggests that eating SPI can lead to a deficiency in a range of nutrients including calcium, magnesium, manganese, copper, iron and zinc.[11] Soya also seems to have the capacity to impair thyroid function,[12] which can lead to diverse symptoms such as weight gain, fatigue and constipation.

Soya has been touted for its cholesterol-reducing properties, though, as we will learn in Chapter 13, this has not been proven

PRIME FUEL

to have broad benefits for health. Soya has also been heavily promoted for its breast cancer-preventative effects. This proposed benefit has been put down to hormone-like molecules found in soya known as 'phytoestrogens'. However, the evidence in this area is mixed, and offers no clear support for the role of dietary phytoestrogens in the prevention of breast cancer.[13]

There is some thought that phytoestrogens have the capacity to impair brain function. One study found a significant statistical relationship between eating tofu and accelerated brain ageing.[14] Soya intake has been associated with impaired semen quality and infertility.[15]

The balance of evidence suggests that soya-based foods should not be emphasized in the diet, particularly in the form of SPI and TVP. Better forms of soya are more natural, less processed, fermented forms of this food such as tempeh, natto and miso.

Summary

- Other than tempeh, natto and miso, which may be eaten in moderation, soya-based foods should be avoided.

Quorn

The main ingredient in Quorn is 'mycoprotein' – derived from a mould organism (*Fusarium venenatum*) that was discovered in soil samples by British scientists in the 1960s. This organism is multiplied en masse in steel containers and then contrived into foods such as 'burgers', 'sausages' and other meat substitutes.

Quorn's manufacturers like to give their product a natural 'flavour' by likening it to mushrooms and truffles. However, according to Professor David Geiser of the Fusarium Research Center at Pennsylvania State University in the USA, drawing parallels between the organism used to make Quorn and mushrooms is like 'calling a rat a chicken because both are animals'.[16] Perhaps not surprisingly, this newfangled food has been linked with adverse reactions, including gastrointestinal complaints.[17]

Like SPI and TVP (see Soya, above), Quorn is a highly processed and quite unnatural food of dubious nutritional merit.

Summary

- Quorn should be avoided.

Nuts and Seeds

Tree-grown nuts such as walnuts, pecans, cashews, hazelnuts and almonds are relatively protein-rich, low-carbohydrate foods. Nuts have a reputation for being fattening, but, as we discovered in Chapter 6 (Low-Fat Fallacy), this is unfounded, and in fact the reverse appears to be generally true.

Nuts are rich in nutrients such as magnesium, potassium, copper, vitamin E and monounsaturated fat – all of which may benefit cardiovascular health. Eating more nuts is associated, albeit in epidemiological studies, with a reduced risk of heart attacks[18] and 'sudden cardiac death'.[19]

Seeds (e.g. pumpkin, sesame, sunflower) have not been formally studied with regard to their effects on health. Because they are nutritionally very similar to nuts, however, we would expect them to have broadly similar benefits for health.

Nuts can be eaten either raw or roasted. Salting of nuts is not an issue unless there is a history of high blood pressure or some suspicion of this.

DO YOUR NUTS

Some people find that eating nuts causes gut problems such as bloating and diarrhoea. The likely culprits here are substances such as lectins, digestion inhibitors and phytates, discussed in Chapter 14 (Grain of Truth). In my experience, such problems occur less frequently with nuts than they do with grains (especially wheat), but they do occur so what to do?

193

Soaking raw nuts and then drying them can neutralise the substances that can cause digestive symptoms. Nuts should be soaked overnight in salty water, after which they should be dried in an oven (on a very low heat and/or with the oven door kept open with a wooden spoon or wine cork). An alternative is to invest in a food dehydrator.

Summary

- Nuts and seeds can be eaten freely and should preferably be eaten in their raw or roasted form. If necessary, they should first be soaked and then dried.

Cooking Oils

Many 'vegetable' oils, such as sunflower, soya and corn oils, are rich in omega-6 fats, a general excess of which exists in the diet. Healthier options include olive oil, macadamia nut oil and avocado oil (all rich in monounsaturated fat) and coconut oil (rich in saturated fat). Coconut oil has the added advantage of being generally stable at a high temperature (therefore good for cooking). It is also rich in what are known as 'medium-chain fatty acids' (including lauric acid and capric acid). These fats have been found to help protect the body from infection from organisms including bacteria, viruses and yeasts.

Sesame oil contains roughly equal amounts of omega-6 and monounsaturated fat, and may be used in moderation.

Summary

- Olive oil, avocado oil and coconut oil may be eaten freely.

- Sesame oil may be eaten in moderation.

- Other vegetable oils should be avoided.

Butter and Margarine

The relative attributes of butter and margarine were explored in Chapter 12 (A Matter of Fat), which revealed butter to be the clear winner. It also tastes better.

Summary

- Butter can be eaten freely.

- Margarine should be avoided.

Dairy Products

Other than butter (see above), the main dairy products are milk, cheese, yoghurt, cream and ice cream.

In Chapter 16 (Sacred Cow), we learned that, overall, dairy products have little value in terms of bone health. We also learned that they are quite common causes of food sensitivity, which can be manifested as a range of symptoms including digestive discomfort and wind, asthma, eczema, nasal/sinus congestion and mucus/catarrh. Milk is generally the worst tolerated of the dairy products (particularly pasteurised milk), and goats' and sheep's products are generally better tolerated than those made from cows' milk. Raw products are generally better tolerated than those that have been pasteurized.

On the positive side, the relatively protein- and fat-rich nature of dairy products such as full-fat yoghurt, cheese and cream is a plus. You may remember from Chapter 16 that, despite the fact that dairy products can stimulate insulin secretion, there is evidence that they can also assist fat loss.

I regard strained (Greek) yoghurt as a good option, as the straining process 'concentrates' the yoghurt (making it more substantial as a food) and also removes some of the sugar. If yoghurt is eaten, I recommend that this is in its *full-fat* version, partly because this improves the satisfaction derived from eating it. 'Fruit' and flavoured yoghurts should be avoided as they usually contain heaps of added sugar and/or artificial sweeteners. Plain yoghurt can be made more tasty and nutritious with foods such as berries, nuts and seeds.

Cheese and full-fat cream can be eaten in moderation.

Ice cream and frozen yoghurt are not recommended, at least partly because of their high sugar content. Frozen yoghurt is often sweetened with agave syrup. Promoted as a healthy sweetening agent, this is in fact loaded with fructose and should be avoided.

Summary

- Milk and ice cream should be avoided.

- Sugary or artificially sweetened yoghurts should be avoided.

- If dairy products are consumed, these should be in their full-fat form.

- Plain, full-fat yoghurt may be eaten freely.

- Cream and cheese can be consumed in moderation.

Grains

Generally speaking, grains such as wheat, oats, rye, barley, rice and corn have high GIs and GLs and are not recommended. Moreover, these foods, even in their wholegrain form, offer little from a nutritional perspective. They are generally less nutritious than fruits and vegetables, and also contain phytates that impair nutrient absorption. Grains are also a common cause of food sensitivity issues.

Summary

- Grains should be avoided.

Foods with Added Sugar

Confectionery, sweet pastries, puddings, biscuits, cakes, doughnuts and the like contain a lot of refined flour (generally high GI) and, often, industrially produced fats, and should be avoided.

One sweet treat that might have some place in the diet is dark chocolate (70 per cent cocoa solids or more). More about this can be found in Chapter 17.

Summary

- Foods with added sugar should be avoided except for dark chocolate, which can be eaten in moderation.

Other Foodstuffs

Food containing artificial sweeteners (see Chapter 19), MSG (see Chapter 17) or partially hydrogenated and trans fat (see Chapter 12) should be avoided. In the UK, there is no legal requirement for manufacturers to declare their products' trans fat content. However, the presence of partially hydrogenated fat in a food is an indication that industrially produced trans fats are likely to be present.

Table 8 provides a summary of the food guidelines contained in this chapter. Just to remind you, 'in moderation' foods are best avoided, but can be eaten when it's difficult to eat from 'eat freely' foods, or on the odd occasion that you just fancy something else.

For better initial results, you might want to start by avoiding 'in moderation' foods as much as possible, and relax this slightly after making progress in losing weight. In general, I recommend having a modest portion of an 'in moderation' food (e.g. a serving of lentils or hunk of cheese as a snack) no more than once a day. In the long term, remember, the aim is to ensure that the bulk (80 per cent or more) of your diet is made up of 'eat freely' foods.

FOOD TO CONSUME IN UNLIMITED QUANTITY	FOOD TO CONSUME IN MODERATION	FOOD TO AVOID
meat (unprocessed) and homemade burgers/patties/meatballs	processed meat e.g. bacon, ham, salami, sausages	
fish (especially oily fish such as salmon, mackerel, herring and sardines) and seafood	tuna, marlin, swordfish	
eggs		
berries, avocado	apples, pears, plums, citrus fruits (mango, pineapple, and banana in more limited quantities)	dried fruit
green vegetables, cauliflower, salad vegetables, onions, tomatoes, mushrooms	squash, pumpkin, carrots, swede, parsnips, sweet potato	white potato
		beans, lentils, peas and peanuts except in small quantities
	fermented soya products such as tempeh, natto and miso	soya milk and soya products based on TVP and SPI
		quorn
	dark chocolate	foods with added sugar such as soft drinks, confectionery, biscuits, cakes, pastries
nuts and seeds		
butter, olive oil, avocado oil, coconut oil	sesame oil	margarine
plain full-fat yoghurt (especially strained)	cream, cheese (goat's and sheep's cheeses preferred)	sweetened yoghurt, milk, ice cream
		foods with added suagr
		grain-based foods such as bread, rice, pasta, breakfast cereals, crackers
		foods containing MSG
		foods containing artificial sweeteners
		foods containing partially hydrogenated fats

Table 8: Summary of food recommendations

ESCAPE THE DIET TRAP

Chapter 19

FLUID THINKING

Effective fat loss and optimal health aren't just about what we eat, but also what we *drink*. In this chapter we'll be taking an in-depth look at the major beverages in the modern-day diet, with a view to assessing their appropriateness with regard to both weight control and wellbeing. We'll start with water, before turning our attention to coffee, tea, fruit juice, soft drinks and alcoholic beverages. As with the preceding chapter, each beverage will be rated as something to drink freely, in moderation or not at all.

Water – the Forgotten Nutrient

The adult human body is about two-thirds water and this fact alone suggests that water has an important part to play in our health and wellbeing. Actually, all of our biochemical, physiological and neurological processes depend to some degree on water. Water, for instance, helps maintain the circulation, and is important for proper functioning of the brain and nervous system, too.

Because water plays a critical role in the body's most fundamental processes, dehydration can manifest itself in myriad ways. Lethargy (of both body and mind) is a common symptom, as are headaches and constipation. For optimal health and wellbeing, it pays to keep topped up with water.

FAT FLUSH?

'Detox' regimes are often recommended as a path to weight loss, and a major component of such regimes is water. While the idea that simply drinking more water might assist in the search for a slimmer body may seem unlikely, there does seem to be scientific evidence to support this.

For example, it has been found that cells that are dehydrated do not take up glucose very efficiently[1] – something that could cause the metabolism to stall. Also, studies show that when the blood is made more dilute, fat release from the fat cells (lipolysis) is enhanced.[2,3] This evidence suggests that there is some support for the notion that keeping well hydrated can assist us in our quest to shed fat.

How Much Water Do We Need?

Our need for water is dependent on many different factors including our propensity to sweat, body size, activity levels, temperature, humidity and how much water might be taken in from, say, fruit and vegetables. It's therefore difficult to make a general recommendation about water intake, but better for us to tune into personal indicators of our state of hydration.

Many people judge their need to drink on thirst. The problem here is that once thirst is sensed, the body can be quite dehydrated. A better gauge is the colour of our urine.[4] Essentially, the paler our urine is, the better our state of hydration.

The aim is to drink enough water to keep urine pale yellow in colour throughout the day.

If our urine colour strays into darker tones and starts to become noticeably odorous, then there's a very good chance we have allowed ourselves to get dehydrated. In such situations, drinking more water generally improves energy levels and sense of wellbeing within about half an hour.

KEEP WATER BY YOU

For many people, the idea of drinking 2 or more litres of water a day seems like quite a feat. The one piece of advice I have about getting plenty of water into the body each day is this: *keep it by you*. When people have water in front of them, they tend to drink a lot more than if they repeatedly need to get it from, say, the fridge or the water cooler at the end of the corridor.

If you're gardening, keep a bottle of water with you. Put a bottle of water on your desk at work and make sure there is water available in meetings. Put a bottle of water in the car and carry one in your briefcase, rucksack or sports bag when you are out and about. If you keep water by you, you're likely to get through decent quantities of it (but if you don't, you probably *won't*).

Summary

- Water may be drunk in volumes large enough to keep urine pale yellow in colour throughout the course of the day.

Herbal and Fruit Teas

Herbal and fruit teas are an alternative to water for those seeking to maintain good levels of hydration throughout the day. In addition, some of these beverages may have some therapeutic benefit for the body. Fennel and peppermint, for instance, may aid digestion, while chamomile can help ensure restful sleep.

Summary

- Herbal and fruit teas can be drunk freely.

Tea

Tea comes in two main forms – black (regular tea) and green. Basically, black tea is made by allowing green tea to undergo oxidation (through fermentation). Both black and green tea contain caffeine and other stimulants, as well as disease-preventative compounds known as polyphenols, which have 'antioxidant' activity. This means they have the capacity to neutralize the effects of damaging, disease-causing molecules called 'free radicals'. In general, green tea contains less caffeine and has more antioxidant capacity than black tea.

Research links drinking black tea with a reduced risk of heart disease, and three or more cups of black tea a day seems to be what is required to enjoy this benefit.[5] Black tea has also been associated with a reduced risk of stroke in men.[6]

Drinking green tea has also been associated with a reduced risk of heart disease.[7] Any benefit that exists here is thought to be, at least in part, due to a 'polyphenol' found in green tea called 'epigallocatechin-3-gallate' (EGCG), which is one of a group of compounds known as 'catechins'. EGCG has also been found to have a number of cancer-preventative actions in the body, including an ability to help deactivation of cancer-causing chemicals (carcinogens). There is evidence to suggest that regular consumption of green tea is associated with a reduced risk of some forms of cancer.[7]

CAN GREEN TEA HELP FAT-BURNING IN THE BODY?

Some research has explored the role that green tea may play in the metabolism of fat in the body. In one study, giving men green tea extract (containing 350 mg of EGCG)[8] was found to enhance fat metabolism by 17 per cent. In another,[9] treating overweight men with 300 mg of EGCG for just two days stimulated the metabolism of fat after a meal. Other research has found that drinking catechin-rich tea regularly for 12 weeks led to significant reductions in body weight, waist size and fat mass compared to drinking low-catechin tea.[10] The catechin content of the 'active' tea was 690 mg a day, which equates to about 5–6 cups of green tea.

In a similar study,[11] individuals were given a daily beverage containing 625 mg of catechins for a period of 12 weeks. Study participants were instructed to undertake three or more hours of moderately intense activity each week. These individuals saw a significant reduction in abdominal fat compared to those consuming a 'control' drink that was not rich in catechins.

A word of caution: there is evidence that green tea components appear to block the action of the chemotherapy drug bortezomib (Velcade).[12] Those taking this drug should consult their doctors regarding green tea use.

Coffee

Coffee has a somewhat unhealthy reputation, and much of this is based on its relatively high caffeine content. On the other hand, coffee is very rich in disease-preventative 'antioxidant' substances including so-called polyphenols. Coffee is actually consistently associated with a reduced risk of diabetes[13–15] and metabolic syndrome.[16] Its consumption is also associated with a reduced risk of stroke.[17,18] Although epidemiological, this evidence is consistent with the fact that coffee contains substances that are beneficial to health.

HIGH LIFE

Coffee and tea contain caffeine and other stimulants that can potentially have adverse effects on health including sleep disturbance. Individuals vary widely in their tolerance to caffeine. Some can feel a distinct 'jolt' from caffeine soon after it is drunk and need to be particularly careful regarding their caffeine

FLUID THINKING

consumption if they want to sleep well. Others can throw back a double espresso after dinner and sleep like babies.

If you feel you are sensitive to caffeine, you might want to consider drinking decaffeinated coffee and tea. Decaffeination processes, however, can involve chemical solvents that are best avoided. More natural, and preferred, forms of decaffeination use water (also known as the 'Swiss' method) or carbon dioxide. Careful reading of labels is required to find appropriate brands.

A word of warning: abrupt withdrawal of caffeine can precipitate a headache (this is a common cause of 'weekend headaches', by the way). The headache normally comes on the day caffeine is eliminated, and dissipates over the next two days or so. Gradual withdrawal of caffeine can prevent any such symptoms.

One to Remember

Some evidence also links coffee drinking with a reduced risk of dementia, including Alzheimer's disease.[19,20] It is possible that the antioxidants in coffee help protect brain cells from the damage wreaked by chemical entities known as 'free radicals'. Also, coffee consumption is associated with a reduced risk of diabetes, and diabetes is a risk factor for dementia. It is also possible that coffee may provide some protection against dementia through its ability to deliver caffeine to the body. One study found that giving caffeine to mice with Alzheimer's disease improved their brain function.[21] Caffeine also reduces the production of the protein beta-amyloid, deposits of which are a hallmark feature in the brains of Alzheimer's sufferers.

THE PRIMAL PRINCIPLE – TEA AND COFFEE

It's hard to imagine our early ancestors sitting around campfires drinking espressos and sipping green tea. However, the main constituent of these drinks is *water*. And let's not forget that coffee comes from a bean and tea from a leaf – both of which occur naturally. While they look and taste different, both tea and coffee are rich in health-promoting substances. When such substances are infused in hot water, it's perhaps not that surprising that the resultant beverages may turn out to have benefits for health.

Summary

- Caffeinated tea and coffee may be drunk in moderation.

- Naturally decaffeinated tea and coffee may be drunk freely.

Sugary Soft Drinks

Sugary soft drinks generally contain sugar in the form of high fructose corn syrup, though in some the predominant sugar is glucose and/or sucrose. We examined the possibly adverse effects of sugar, including fructose, in Chapter 15 (Sweet and Sour). One major problem with sugary drinks is how available the sugar is to the body. Also, these drinks allow a lot of sugar to be consumed very quickly, compounding the problem.

Summary

- Sugary soft drinks should be avoided.

Artificially Sweetened Beverages

Because artificial sweeteners contain virtually no calories, they are therefore often promoted as a 'healthy' alternative to sugar, particularly for those looking to lose weight. In Chapter 17 (Appetite for Change), we reviewed evidence that artificial sweeteners have the potential to stimulate the appetite, and Chapter 15 (Sweet and Sour) reviewed a study in which feeding animals artificially sweetened food led to them eating more and getting fatter.

In addition to these weight-related effects, there is evidence linking artificial sweeteners to health risks. In one study,[22] Italian researchers fed aspartame in a variety of doses to rats in the long term. Rats consuming aspartame at doses lower than those permitted for humans had significantly increased risk of several forms of cancer. Aspartame has also been linked with a range of adverse effects on health, including headaches,[23,24] and depression.[25]

The manufacturers of aspartame, and the trade organizations and scientists that represent them, will, of course, point to plenty of studies that apparently vouch for aspartame's safety. But there are also plenty that suggest it poses genuine hazards to health. A review of such studies[26] shows that while every single industry funded study concludes that aspartame is safe, the vast majority of independently funded research and reports identify aspartame as a potential problem. I advise avoiding artificial sweeteners.

Summary

- Artificially sweetened drinks should be avoided.

Fruit Juice and Smoothies

Fruit juices are often seen as healthy drinks that are roughly equivalent, in nutritional terms, to whole fruit. However, in juicing a fruit many of the nutritious elements, especially fibre, are left behind. Also, the sugar concentration of fruit juices (even unsweetened ones) is often the same or even higher than that of sugary soft drinks.

Smoothies based on mashed, whole fruit are perhaps healthier than fruit juice. However, they are still intensely sugary and need to be consumed with care. I advise that they are drunk in moderation, and not at all until you are near to achieving your weight and health goals. Moderation is also important for individuals with known insulin resistance, metabolic syndrome or Type 2 diabetes. Another reason for avoiding smoothies is that they are very sweet, and can perpetuate a desire or 'need' for sweetness in the diet.

Summary

- Fruit juice should be avoided.

- Smoothies may be consumed in moderation.

Alcohol

Alcoholic beverages are generally a source of carbohydrate which, remember, is a prime driver of weight gain. Perhaps unsurprisingly, several studies show that higher alcohol intakes are associated with greater body weight. Many studies have also found an association between higher alcohol intakes and increased risk of abdominal obesity.[27–29]

For a given amount of alcohol, beer contains much more carbohydrate than wine (they're not called 'beer bellies' for nothing). Red wine contains, generally speaking, less carbohydrate than white. So, if your goal is to lose fat effectively, drink as little as possible, and when you do drink, perhaps limit yourself to a glass of red wine with your evening meal.

However, in certain circumstances spirits might be an even better option than red wine. While they typically have an unhealthy reputation, in reality they contain very little carbohydrate for a given amount of alcohol. The real issue with spirits is usually any mixer that accompanies them. Fruit juice, tonic water, lemonade and cola will all provide much sugar and/ or artificial sweetener.

Vodka and soda with a twist of lime (or even a splash of lime cordial) represents a good option all round for those who like it. Vodka has the advantage of being a generally pure spirit that is unlikely to induce much in the way of a hangover the following day.

Is Moderate Drinking Healthy?

Moderate drinking is often promoted as something that is 'healthy', essentially because of its links with a reduced risk of heart disease. One problem with this epidemiological research, however, is that it sometimes fails to consider confounding factors that can cause the drinking of alcohol to appear healthier than it actually is. For instance, non-drinkers at increased risk of heart disease may be reformed alcoholics, or may have stopped drinking because they've been diagnosed with heart disease. A better assessment would include only lifelong teetotallers in the non-drinking group.

Another major flaw in much alcohol research is that it has often focused only on *heart disease*. Alcohol has been linked with adverse effects on health including an increased risk of cancer. It makes sense, therefore, to assess alcohol's relationship with *overall risk of death*.

When researchers have focused on overall mortality, a slightly different picture from the image of alcohol being a 'healthy tipple' emerges. One study found that in men up to the age of thirty-four, the optimal amount of alcohol to drink was none at all.[30] In this study there seemed to be some benefits from alcohol consumption later in life – the optimal intake being about 1 unit a day. As a sometime drinker myself, I take no satisfaction in imparting this news, but it seems that the 'benefits' of drinking alcohol have been overstated.

EASY WAYS TO DRINK LESS WITHOUT SACRIFICE

While I think the 'benefits' of alcohol have been somewhat overplayed, I am also of the belief that not everything that passes our lips need be explicitly healthy. There are obviously reasons for consuming foodstuffs that have nothing to do with health. However, the fact remains that any more than very moderate drinking is likely to jeopardize weight-loss efforts and may harm health, so taking steps to control alcohol consumption without any sense of sacrifice or deprivation makes sense.

One tactic that works well is to match each alcoholic drink (e.g. glass of wine) with a glass of water. This usually leads to less wine being drunk, and also dilutes any negative effects alcohol may have. Any additional water drunk here is likely to be broadly beneficial to the body, too.

Another way of containing alcohol consumption is to avoid dehydration and thirst before starting drinking. It stands to reason that if alcohol is being drunk, more will be consumed if you're thirsty.

While you're avoiding thirst, I advise avoiding hunger, too. I've found this to be a prime driver of drinking, particularly early in the evening. Even unconsciously, many individuals use alcohol as a replacement for food when they are hungry, particularly if their blood sugar level has taken a dive.

Sour Grapes

Red wine, more than any other form of alcohol, has often been recommended as 'healthy'. Much scientific research has been focused on a constituent in red grapes known as 'resveratrol', the actions of which in the body would help to explain the suggested benefits of red wine for the heart. However, a close look at the evidence reveals that wine drinkers, compared to those who generally drink beer and spirits, for example, tend to have healthier diets and to smoke less, too.[31–33] These studies actually show it's not the red wine *per se*, but these other factors associated with drinking red wine, that probably account for its apparent 'benefits'.

Summary

- Alcohol should be drunk in moderation.

- Because of their generally low carbohydrate content, red wine and spirits are preferred over white wine and beer.

WHAT DOES 'MODERATION' MEAN?

The same 'in moderation' rules apply to drinks as to food: wherever possible, opt for drinks such as water, herbal and fruit teas, and naturally decaffeinated tea or coffee. In the initial stages of changing your diet, avoid doing this more than once a day. In the long term you can relax this, but aim to ensure that at least 80 per cent of your fluid intake comes from beverages that can be consumed in unlimited quantity.

BEVERAGES TO CONSUME IN UNLIMITED QUANTITY	BEVERAGES TO CONSUME IN MODERATION	BEVERAGES TO AVOID
water		
herb and fruit teas		
naturally decaffeinated coffee and tea	caffeinated coffee and tea	
	smoothies (small quantities only)	fruit juice
	red wine, spirits	sugary and artificially sweetened soft drinks
		white wine, beer, cider

Table 9: Summary of beverage recommendations

Chapter 20

MAKE A MEAL OF IT

So far in this book we have looked at the science of healthy weight loss and translated that into food recommendations. Here, we're going to convert this information into recommendations for actual meals and snacks. So, what to eat?

Breakfast

Many people find that without breakfast it can be difficult for them to make healthy choices during the rest of the day. For some, though not all, there's something about a decent breakfast that can 'hold' the appetite later on and make choosing a good lunch and dinner relatively easy.

These days, speed and convenience are priorities in the morning for many people. One option that works well here is a yoghurt-based breakfast. I recommend full-fat Greek yoghurt as the base, to which can be added berries (e.g. fresh strawberries, blueberries and raspberries or frozen berries that have been defrosted) and nuts (e.g. chopped almonds and walnuts). Certain berries (e.g. blackberries) can be a bit tart, so you might allow yourself a faint drizzle of honey. Other than the honey, there's no need to limit quantities at all.

One of the good things about this breakfast is that it travels well. Those who travel to work may leave home before they are even hungry. The yoghurt mix can be taken in a container to be eaten en route to work or even in the workplace.

Another option that can be enjoyed outside the home is an omelette or frittata. Goat's cheese and chorizo or goat's cheese and spinach work well here. Yet another is to make 'breadless Scotch eggs' ahead of time. All this entails is wrapping minced pork (or other meat) around a small hard-boiled egg, leaving it in the fridge to chill, then shallow- or deep-fry it.

At the weekend, I generally recommend cooked breakfasts/ brunches. Smoked salmon and scrambled eggs are a good combination, or even just poached eggs with fried mushrooms and tomato. Wilted spinach can make a good accompaniment here, too. Just wash some spinach leaves, shake them dry and add to a heated frying pan or saucepan and keep moving the spinach until it has softened. Add some butter (if you like) and serve.

If you're feeling a little more adventurous you might whip up a Hollandaise sauce. There's a quick and easy way of doing this: take a couple of egg yolks, add some lemon juice and whip with an electric hand blender while you add very hot melted butter little by little.

A 'full English' is another option. Cooked breakfasts are a very good idea if you're staying at a hotel (just don't eat the bread and pastries on offer).

Some people simply don't need much food in the morning, and find a couple of handfuls of nuts and maybe a piece of fruit is all they require, say, in the mid- or late-morning. As long as someone on such a regime maintains good energy and brain function throughout the morning and does not end up famished by lunchtime, there's nothing wrong with this at all.

Lunch

If you're at home for lunch, as long as you have the right food to hand, there are plenty of easy options. Examples include:

- Omelette and salad.

- Grilled chops or fish with salad.

- Reheated stew or casserole.

- Bolognese sauce eaten either just with grated parmesan and some salad or on a bed of cabbage 'tagliatelle' (shredded and steamed cabbage).

- Meaty fresh soup (shop-bought or home-made).

Often the biggest challenge for lunch eaters is how to avoid sandwiches when they're not at home. One alternative is salad, and many sandwich bars and shops will have these ready-made. If you're not vegetarian, I suggest making a conscious effort to include meat or fish here, as it will help ensure the salad sustains you throughout the afternoon. If you are vegetarian, look for salads that contain egg, cheese or avocado, for much-needed protein and fat.

Sandwich bars and the like often offer soups at lunch, usually both meat and vegetable. Again, unless you have good reason not to, I suggest opting for the meat variety.

Remember, it's very important not to be too hungry before lunch: having a contained appetite makes avoiding bread and other carb-rich accompaniments (such as chocolate, cereal bars and crisps) easy.

Bear in mind, too, that what you eat at lunch does not necessarily need to get you through to dinner – if you get hungry again you can always eat some nuts (and perhaps a piece of fruit and a couple of squares of dark chocolate) in the late afternoon or early evening.

MAKE A MEAL OF IT

WOT, NO DESSERTS?

Desserts by their very nature are sweet, and that generally means the presence of lots of sugar or artificial sweetener, neither of which has much of a place in a truly healthy diet. Plus, eating desserts further accustoms the taste buds to sweet foods, which itself can perpetuate a desire for them. In the long run, it can be easier (not to mention healthier) to cut out dessert, apart from odd occasions such as part of a celebratory meal or if you find yourself in a particularly swanky restaurant and simply want to indulge yourself. Any treat of this nature should be savoured and is nothing to feel guilty or regretful about. Just put its eating into the context of your diet as a whole and see it pale into insignificance.

Dinner

The lunch options referred to above all work as dinners. Key, once again, is to think 'primal'. Another quick and easy option is cold meat (e.g. cold chicken, cold roast beef) and/or fish (e.g. smoked salmon, smoked trout, peppered mackerel), served with salad or crudités, perhaps with some hummus and olives. For those who normally round off their evening meal with dessert (e.g. ice cream, yoghurt), I suggest a couple of squares of dark chocolate.

If you're eating in a restaurant, and are opting for two courses, then something salad-based (e.g. smoked duck salad, smoked salmon salad, tomato, avocado and mozzarella salad) would be a good place to start. Follow this with some meat or fish with vegetables (hold the potatoes). If you're vegetarian, think about something like a roast vegetable stack and salad or just a nice big salad, preferably with some avocado and cheese for additional protein and fat.

As usual, make sure you don't sit down to eat too hungry. I stress this as there's a tendency for people to hold back on food when they know they're going out to dinner to 'compensate' for the expected calorie onslaught to come. The irony is, it's going hungry in the day that usually brings about excessive eating. Ensuring your appetite is under reasonable control when eating in a restaurant is what takes the challenge out of turning down things like bread, risotto, pasta or a side order of chips.

Some people are concerned about eating too late. Personally, I think the real problem is not eating too late, it's eating *too much too late*. There's an argument for eating smaller evening meals than we traditionally do. Appetite control is key here, again, and eating well during the day and grabbing a snack in the late afternoon/early evening can be critical.

Snacks

Fruit is often recommended as the healthy snack of choice, but I generally advise against this. As I mentioned in Chapter 17 (Appetite for Change), fruit often fails to satisfy the appetite properly (it's also very sugar-rich and not ideal for some people).

Better options for snacks include:

- Nuts.

- Seeds (e.g. toasted pumpkin seeds).

- Olives.

- Biltong (air-dried meat).

- Cold meat (e.g. roast beef, chicken).

- Hard-boiled eggs.

- Breadless Scotch eggs.

OUT OF SIGHT ...

One concern some individuals have is how many nuts they can eat as a snack and what constitutes a 'portion'. You'll notice that throughout this book I recommend no specific serving sizes, amounts or weights of food. That's because as long as individuals have not allowed themselves to get too hungry, and as long as they're eating real, nutritious, sustaining food, then overeating is not a problem. In other words, individuals can rely on their sense of satiety to regulate intake automatically and without any need for conscious restriction.

However, in theory it is possible to overeat things like nuts, particularly when you are distracted. Sitting in front of the TV or the laptop it's quite possible to polish off a sizeable bag of nuts without even really being conscious of this. This sort of 'mindless eating' can lead some to consume more food than they need to.

One simple remedy for this is for snacks such as nuts to be kept available, so that they can be eaten when required, but not *visible*. You should know they're there should you need them, but you can't see them and they're certainly not, say, in front of you *on* your desk or in a big bowl perched on the arm of your sofa.

Ideal storage places would be inside a kitchen cupboard, a desk drawer, a handbag, briefcase or laptop bag, or the glove compartment in a car. Now, if you get peckish, you're at liberty to take some nuts and eat them. I recommend tipping a few into the palm of the hand and returning the bag to where it's normally stored. If you're still hungry after a while, go back and take some more. It's unlikely you'll do this, though, unless genuine hunger and peckishness remain.

Keeping food out of sight is usually enough to prevent mindless eating.

ESCAPE THE DIET TRAP

TAKEAWAY TAKE-HOME MESSAGES

Takeaways do not need to be a nutritional disaster area. It is possible to enjoy them and still eat relatively healthily. The first rule is not to be too hungry when you are ordering. Grabbing a takeaway late on the way home from work when you had lunch eight or more hours ago, or when staggering back from the pub, are not situations that lend themselves to making healthy choices.

Ordering a takeaway for you (and perhaps others) on a weekend night in a non-famished state is much more compatible with healthy eating. The trick is to think 'primal'. So, for instance, if Indian food is the order of the day you might opt for a meat- or prawn-based curry, or tikka dish, plus vegetables, say, in the form of sag paneer (Indian cheese and spinach) and some dhal (lentils). If you're not too hungry, you won't miss the rice and naan bread that can really do the damage. If Chinese food is in the offing, perhaps opt for a beef, prawn or chicken dish (e.g. beef with ginger, spicy prawns, chicken with cashew nuts) and some stir-fried vegetables. Again, hold the rice.

If you do happen to find yourself hungry late at night and in need of something to eat, I'd suggest a shish kebab – lamb, raw vegetables and not too much in the way of an unhealthy carb load (bread) – won't do a great deal of harm in the grand scheme of things.

GET READY FOR READY MEALS

There's a strong theme running through this book that the diet should be made up, as much as possible, of natural, unprocessed foods. However, we don't always have the time to cook from fresh ingredients, and this is one reason why some of us may be tempted by convenience foods and ready meals. Many of these, for example microwaveable lasagne, are never going to get you closer to your fat loss and health goals. However, that does not mean that all ready meals are off-limits.

A ready meal comprising a piece of fish or meat with vegetables is, to all intents and purposes, no more processed than something you might prepare at home. It might have a bit more salt than you would normally use, but it's essentially quite *unprocessed* – just food prepared in a factory rather than your kitchen. As with takeaways, the trick is to stick to ready meals that are made from primal ingredients. Such meals are a good compromise between healthy eating and convenience.

Typical Eating Plans

Here are some examples of what a typical day's eating might look like. The snacks are entirely optional – if you don't need them to keep your appetite under control, don't eat them. Most people find when eating this way that they have little or no need for a mid-morning snack, but that one in the late afternoon often has tremendous value.

These eating plans demonstrate how putting into practice the dietary suggestions here may look in the real world. They can be used to inspire your own choices, based on your personal food preferences.

Weekday options:

Breakfast – yoghurt, nut and berry mix (eaten at home, on the way to work, or at work)
Snack – raw or roasted nuts
Lunch – crayfish and avocado salad (shop-bought)
Snack – raw or roasted nuts and some dark chocolate
Dinner – home-made beefburger and salad

Breakfast – 1–2 breadless Scotch eggs (eaten on way to work or at work)
Snack – raw or roasted mixed nuts
Lunch – reheated chilli con carne and salad (no rice)
Snack – mixed nuts and a piece of fruit (e.g. apple or pear)

Dinner – grilled salmon with tomato, onion and coriander salad

Breakfast – chorizo and goat's cheese omelette (either hot or cold)
Snack – raw or roasted nuts
Lunch – meaty soup (shop-bought)
Snack – raw or roasted nuts and some dark chocolate
Dinner – grilled fish with salad or buttered green vegetables

Weekend options:

Breakfast/brunch – cooked breakfast (e.g. smoked salmon and
    poached eggs, bacon and eggs)
Snack – raw or roasted nuts and a piece of fruit
Lunch/snack – cheese, celery and cold meats
Dinner – meat casserole and vegetables

Breakfast/brunch – scrambled eggs and smoked salmon with
    mushrooms
Snack – raw or roasted nuts and a piece of fruit
Lunch – cheese, celery and cold meats
Snack – raw or roasted nuts
Dinner – seafood stew and salad

Breakfast/brunch – poached eggs with wilted spinach and ham
    (optional)
Snack – raw or roasted nuts
Lunch – salmon salad Niçoise
Snack – raw or roasted mixed nuts and dark chocolate
Dinner – roast chicken, beef or lamb with vegetables

PASS THE SALT

When people scale back their consumption of carbohydrate, their
insulin levels will generally tumble. This is a good thing, but it can
have biochemical repercussions that we need to be aware of and
manage.

One of insulin's effects is to reduce the rate at which sodium is excreted through the kidneys. With more sodium in the system, there will be a tendency for the body to retain fluid, too. This is one reason why individuals eating a carbohydrate-rich diet can be somewhat 'waterlogged', one sign of which is swelling in the feet and lower legs.

When carbohydrate intake is contained and insulin levels drop, the kidneys ramp up their excretion of sodium, which takes water with it. This means that some people find themselves urinating more than they usually do for a few days, and it can cause sodium levels to drop significantly too. Also, if you've moved away from processed foods, sodium intake will probably drop, compounding the issue.

In some people this can lead to symptoms such as fatigue, headache, cramp or light-headedness.

One way of countering this is to make a point of adding salt to your food during cooking or at the table. Obviously, you don't want to do this to the extent that you're finding the taste of your food brackish, but, up to this point, generally the more salt you add the better. Another strategy is to add some salt to your drinking water. Add enough so that the water tastes faintly salty.

Over time, your body will have the opportunity to adjust to your new diet and restore sodium balance. I find people can back off the salt over 2–4 weeks without any ill effect.

Chapter 21

AFFIRMATIVE ACTION

The earlier chapters of *Escape the Diet Trap* explain why eating less rarely works for the long-term shedding of fat. You may well remember from the first chapter, though, that adding exercise to a restrictive diet does little to improve matters. In this chapter, we're going to explore *why* this is.

This is not to say that exercise has no value – there's little doubt that it can be beneficial for general health and wellbeing. Also, 'resistance' exercise can do wonders to enhance the strength and the appearance of the body. Practical advice about how to benefit from exercise using realistic, sustainable approaches will be found in this chapter, too.

Energy to Burn?

The most commonly recommended form of exercise for weight control is aerobic activity – essentially, forms of exercise that can be sustained for prolonged periods of time including walking, running, cycling and swimming. By increasing the amount of calories burned by the body, aerobic exercise theoretically enhances weight loss. Yet, as we learned in Chapter 1, regular exercise has only marginal benefits here (a loss of about 1 kg) when used as an adjunct to dietary change. Can science explain why the apparent return on our investment here is so small?

Imagine taking the oft-quoted advice to get 30 minutes of exercise five times a week. A 30-minute jog, say, will burn about 300 calories. However, just sitting watching television will burn about 50 calories in the same time, so the *additional* calorie burn for half an hour's worth of jogging is 250 calories. Do this five times in a week, and you'll have burned a total of about 1,250 calories.

Now, assuming that *all* those calories will be lost in the form of fat (certainly not assured), and that you don't eat more as a result of expending more energy (more on this in a moment), then your jogging endeavours over the week will lead to a loss of about third of a pound of fat (remember, each pound of fat contains about 3,500 calories). Simple maths reveals one of the fundamental problems with using aerobic exercise for weight loss: it just doesn't burn *that* many calories.

Some claim that additional calories are burned *after* exercise, too, and this needs to be factored into our assessment. There is some truth in this, but the effect is relatively small and unlikely to lead to any meaningful weight loss. For moderately intense activity lasting up to an hour, fat metabolism over the next 24 hours is essentially the same as when no exercise had been taken.[1]

Another barrier to losing weight through aerobic exercise is the hunger it can bring on[2] – hence the expression 'working up an appetite'. Undoing the calorie deficit induced by a 30-minute jog doesn't take much, either (three plain digestive biscuits or a pint and a half of beer will do it). Some people also reward themselves with food after exercise (you know who you are …).

Something else that may explain the lack of effectiveness of exercise in weight loss concerns the fact that when individuals take more exercise they naturally tend to become more sedentary in other areas of their lives.[3–6] Prolonged exercise can also lead to sustained rises in levels of the hormone cortisol, which, as we learned in Chapter 6 (Low-Fat Fallacy) predisposes to fat gain, and to abdominal obesity in particular.

ESCAPE THE DIET TRAP

Put all these potential effects of exercise together and it's obvious why using traditional exercise for weight loss can be an uphill struggle.

COULD POOR WEIGHT-LOSS RESULTS FROM EXERCISE BE DOWN TO MUSCLE GAIN?

One explanation for the failure of exercise to induce weight loss could be that exercise builds muscle, which offsets the weight that is lost due to loss of fat. However, the aerobic exercises deployed in such exercises don't build significant quantities of muscle. The logical conclusion is, therefore, that aerobic exercise is quite ineffective in shifting fat.

Things Are Not Always as They Seem

Some people find it hard to get their head round the fact that aerobic exercise is not particularly effective for weight loss, even when faced with all the facts. One reason for this is our experience of seeing physically fit and active individuals who are clearly *lean*. Look at any elite long-distance runner or Tour de France cyclist and you're probably getting a glimpse of what it's like to have a single-digit body fat percentage (that's *very* low). The automatic thought process is that *exercise causes leanness.*

However, could it that individuals who are naturally lean are simply more likely to end up as elite long-distance runners or cyclists? In other words, might their natural leanness cause certain people to be more active, rather than the other way round?

Far-fetched though this may seem, there's actually some evidence for this. In one piece of research, the relationship between physical activity and body fatness in children over a 3-year period was assessed.[7] It was found that the more sedentary children were, the more fat they carried.

This is all to be expected, but because the study was conducted over a prolonged period the researchers were able to gauge whether sedentary behaviour *preceded* weight gain. Actually, it did not. In reality, children accumulated fat first, and *then* became more sedentary. The authors noted that this finding 'may explain why attempts to tackle childhood obesity by promoting PA [physical activity] have been largely unsuccessful'.

What About Weight Maintenance?

Aerobic exercise may not be very effective for weight loss, but could it help *maintain* your leaner condition? The evidence shows that successful maintenance of weight loss through exercise requires a considerable amount of time and effort: one major review found that 60–90 minutes of daily activity is required to increase substantially someone's chances of preventing weight regain after weight loss.[8] That's a lot of time spent exercising just to stand still from a weight perspective.

Let's Get Physical

All this talk about how ineffective exercise generally is for weight control may give you the impression that I'm somewhat anti-exercise. Nothing could be further from the truth. I don't, though, want to perpetuate the commonly held myth about the value of aerobic exercise in shedding pounds. In the next chapter, however, I'll be describing a form of exercise that does seem to be genuinely effective for fat loss, and with relatively brief sessions, too.

While aerobic exercise might not help much with weight loss, it does seem to have the capacity to help reduce the risk of chronic disease and enhance physical and psychological wellbeing.

Take a Walk

One form of aerobic exercise that I think has particular merit is walking. Some people take the view (as I once did) that walking is not strenuous enough to benefit health and fitness. The evidence suggests otherwise.

For example, in one study individuals were instructed to walk briskly for 30 minutes three or five times a week.[9] They could if they wanted break the 30 minutes down into periods of no less than 10 minutes each. Other individuals in this study were not given any walking instructions, and therefore acted as a 'control' or 'inactive' group against whom the results of the 'walkers' could be compared. The research was conducted over a 12-week period.

The walkers saw improvements in fitness, systolic blood pressure (the higher value of the two blood pressure measurements) and an average reduction in waist circumference of more than an inch. Remember, all these benefits can come from nothing more strenuous than walking.

WALKING CAN BOOST BRAIN FUNCTION

Another aspect of health for which exercise may have benefits is brain function. In one study, a group of sedentary middle-aged and elderly individuals had their brain function assessed, and were then randomized (allotted by chance) to one of two exercise regimes: walking (at their own pace) for 40 minutes, three times a week, or regular stretching and toning exercises.[10]

Twelve months later, compared to those who had been stretching and toning, those on the walking regime saw improvements in cognitive tests, especially those relating to what are called 'executive control tasks' (e.g. planning, scheduling, dealing with ambiguity and multi-tasking). It is these skills, by the way, that tend to take a bit of a hit as we age.

225

How Hard Should You Work?

It is generally accepted that exercise needs to be of a certain intensity for you to get any meaningful benefit from it. The heart rate is one way to gauge exercise intensity. Theoretically, the heart rate has a maximum value that is approximately 220 minus a person's age. Benefits are thought to be had from exercising at an intensity equating to 60–75 per cent of the maximum heart rate.

For example, 70 per cent maximum heart rate for a fifty-year-old would equate to $0.7 \times (220 - 45) = $ about 120 beats per minute. If you're not going to check your pulse or use a heart-rate monitor, then aim for a level of intensity where you are somewhat breathless but still able to conduct a conversation. If you can sing (should you want to), you're probably not working hard enough.

As long as walking is genuinely brisk, it's likely that you will be able to exercise at an appropriate intensity. If you find you can't, you might want to consider other forms of activity such as running, cycling or rowing.

How Much Is Enough?

My advice would be to aim for about half an hour's worth of exercise on most days of the week – let's call that a total of about 3 hours of exercise per week. Seems like a lot? It's actually less than 2 per cent of your time.

However busy we may be, most of us could quite easily find time to exercise. Here are a few suggestions:

- Avoid turning the television on in the evening and reduce television viewing time generally.

- Get up earlier (going to bed a bit earlier is the secret here).

- Avoid checking and reading emails incessantly: aim for 1–3 checks at predetermined times each day. If required, set an auto-responder detailing the times you will be checking emails, and how you can be contacted if something is really urgent.

- Avoid spending hours aimlessly surfing the internet.

- Don't buy a newspaper – very rarely will anything important be missed by not getting your daily fix of print media.

- Schedule exercise into the day – at the start of every day or week, plan where your activity is going to go, put it in your diary and commit to it as you would a meeting or appointment.

Is It OK to Split Exercise Up?

Some studies have explored whether the benefits of exercise are still there if, say, a continuous 30 minutes of exercise are split up into smaller periods. The good news is that the benefits are just the same. For example, in one study, three 10-minute sessions of exercise a day improved blood fat (triglyceride) and blood pressure levels as much as a continuous 30-minute session of walking.[11]

In another study, women exercised for a total of 30 minutes each day, several times a week. For one group these 30 minutes comprised one continuous session; for another it was made up of two 15-minute sessions over the course of the day; for another still, it was divided into three 10-minute sessions. All three groups saw similar improvement in measures of fitness.[12]

The evidence shows that getting exercise in bite-sized and more manageable chunks is essentially as beneficial as more extended periods of exercise.

Step Up Your Walking with a Pedometer

Pedometers are small, usually inexpensive, battery-operated devices that are worn on the belt and are used to count steps. There is evidence that using a pedometer encourages higher levels of activity, especially when someone is set a daily target of steps to be taken in a day. Overall, pedometer use appears to increase walking volume by more than a quarter.[13] That, I think, is a good return on the few quid spent buying one.

AFFIRMATIVE ACTION

Offer Some Resistance

Apart from aerobic exercise, the other major form of exercise is known as 'resistance exercise'. Resistance exercise is distinct from aerobic exercises such as jogging and swimming in that it's harder work, and is therefore something that cannot be sustained for extended periods. The intensity of resistance exercise is what gives it the potential to improve the strength and tone of muscles in a way aerobic exercise simply can't. Lifting weights is an example of resistance exercise, though 'free' exercises such as press-ups and sit-ups count, too.

DOES RESISTANCE EXERCISE MIX WITH A HIGH-PROTEIN DIET?

There is evidence that a high-protein diet, coupled with resistance exercise, can be quite a powerful tool for shedding fat. In one study, two diets (one higher in protein than the other) were tried in a group of overweight and obese individuals with Type 2 diabetes.[14] The breakdown of these two diets in terms of calories contributed by carbohydrate, protein and fat respectively were:

- Conventional diet – 53:19:26

- Higher protein diet – 43:33:22

Each group was also split into two, with only one of them engaging in resistance exercise 3 times a week. The study lasted 16 weeks.

Individuals who did the best were those who ate the higher protein diet and did resistance exercise as well. These individuals lost an average of 11.1 kg of fat and 13.7 cm off their waists. In comparison, non-exercising individuals eating a lower protein diet lost an average of 6.4 kg of fat and 8.2 cm off their waists.

Diminishing Losses

When individuals lose weight, there's always the risk that, in addition to shedding fat, they may also lose some muscle. Perhaps not surprisingly, resistance exercise has been found to mitigate this.

In one study, a group of individuals was put on a calorie-restricted diet. The group was then divided into three. One group engaged in resistance exercise, a second engaged in aerobic exercise, while the third just dieted. All groups lost weight, though the resistance-training group lost significantly *less* muscle.[15]

The authors of a review of how best to preserve muscle mass and metabolic rate during weight loss highlight the importance of resistance-training.[16] They also make the point that consuming adequate amounts of protein plays a key role here, too.

Of course, another reason for working your muscles is to get them – and yourself – *looking* better. Resistance exercise plays a huge role here.

A Complete Workout in 12 Minutes

It is possible to improve the look and condition of the body significantly, quite quickly and easily, and with relatively low time investment, too. It's suitable for men and women, and does not run the risk of causing the 'bulking up' that some, particularly women, are keen to avoid.

What follows is a 12-minute resistance exercise-based regime that requires very little special equipment and can be performed at home in an area no bigger than a beach towel. The session is actually made up of two 6-minute sections. The first 6 minutes focus on resistance exercises for the upper body. The second 6 minutes are designed to work the legs with a mix of resistance and aerobic exercises.

SPECIAL EQUIPMENT

There are really only two pieces of equipment you need to consider purchasing:

1. Dyna-Band (or something similar)

Dyna-Bands are essentially giant, wide elastic bands, a few feet in length. They come in different colours, each of which denotes a different resistance. One of the great things about this exercise aid is that it is small and light, and therefore perfect for people who travel or are on the road a lot and want to maintain their exercise regime wherever they are.

2. Dumbbells

A set of dumbbells can be a great investment. Go for a set in which the amount of weight can be varied. These are obviously not for packing in your hand luggage, but a very useful piece of equipment if you're planning to exercise at home.

Start Slowly

The aim with these exercises is to do them continuously for a minute (or as long as you can reasonably manage). If you are out of condition and new to resistance exercise, start with relatively low loads. Choose your Dyna-Band resistance and vary the length of slack accordingly. With the dumbbells, start with relatively light weights and build up over time.

The First 6 Minutes

The first 6 minutes of the session are divided into one-minute blocks, each of which is designed to work a major muscle or muscle group. These are:

1. Chest.

2. Back.

3. Shoulders.

4. Biceps.

5. Triceps.

6. Abdominals.

HOW HARD SHOULD I WORK?

Your ultimate aim is to keep consistent 'form' for each exercise for the whole minute. At the same time, at the end of the minute you should be struggling to perform additional repetitions. Adjust the dumbbell weight or the tension in the Dyna-Band (if relevant), as well as the speed of repetitions, accordingly. As you progress, you can increase these variables to add to your workload.

Full press-ups (see below) are quite hard to do. You may want to start with less intensive versions (half press-up or box press-up) of this exercise to begin with, graduating to full press-ups in time if this is appropriate.

1. Chest

Press-ups

Press-ups exercise and strengthen several muscles including the pectorals (chest), the deltoids (around the shoulders) and triceps (at the back of the upper arm). They also work muscles at the side of the chest wall and in the back.

There's a choice of three here:

- Full press-up – keep your hips and knees straight. Your hands should be directly under your shoulders. Lower your body by bending your elbows until your chest is about 10 cm/4 inches from the floor. Push up again. In addition to exercising the muscles listed above, full press-ups count as a 'core stability' exercise, meaning that it helps strengthen muscles in and around the abdomen, lower back and pelvis.

- Half press-up – similar to full press-ups, but the knees are on the ground set back behind the hips.

- Box press-up – similar to the half, but the knees are directly under the hips.

You might want to put a folded towel under your knees if performing the half and box press-ups.

2. Back

One-armed rows

This exercise is designed to exercise muscles in the back, principally *latissimus dorsi* (found in the flanks), and rhomboids (which run from the inner shoulder blade to the spine). It also exercises the upper arm.

To perform a one-armed row, stand left side on to a sofa or bed and put your left knee on the sofa/bed. Lean forward and place your left hand on the sofa/bed. Keep your right foot on the floor. Take a dumbbell in your right hand with your arm extended vertically. Pull the dumbbell up to your armpit, pause for a moment, and lower the dumbbell again in a controlled fashion. Repeat for 30 seconds, and then reverse your position to do another 30 seconds with your left arm.

This exercise can be performed with a Dyna-Band, which should be trapped under the right foot when exercising the right arm, and the left foot when exercising the left arm.

3. Shoulders

Shoulder press

The shoulder press principally works the deltoid muscle, which is the major muscle in the shoulder at the top of the arm.

To perform the shoulder press, sit comfortably in a steady and firm chair with your back straight. Take dumbbells in both hands and hold them in front of your chest with your palms facing forward. Steadily lift the dumbbells above your head, pause briefly, and return the dumbbells in a controlled fashion to the front of your chest.

This exercise can be performed using a Dyna-Band. Sit on the Dyna-Band and take the ends in each hand. Alternatively, you can perform the exercise while standing with the Dyna-Band trapped under both your feet. You may need to tie two Dyna-Bands together to make them long enough.

4. Biceps

Biceps curls

The biceps is the major muscle at the front of the upper arm. To perform biceps curls, stand with a dumbbell in each hand and let your arms hang, palms facing forward. Lift both dumbbells to your shoulders, pause briefly and lower again in a controlled fashion.

This exercise can be performed using a Dyna-Band, in which case the Dyna-Band should be trapped under both feet.

5. Triceps

Triceps dips

The triceps is the major muscle at the back of the upper arm. You will need a chair for this exercise. Place the front of the chair behind you. Put your palms on the seat of the chair with your fingers pointing forward. Bend your knees and keep your feet flat on the floor. Take your weight on your arms and slowly bend your elbows to 90 degrees, lowering your hips towards the floor. Push back up again. Keep your back straight and close to the chair throughout this exercise.

If you do not have access to a chair or something similar and are unable to perform this exercise, don't worry – press-ups (see above) will give your triceps a decent workout, too.

6. Abdominals

Sit-ups

Lie with your back flat on the floor, knees bent and feet flat. Place your right hand on your right thigh and place your left hand behind your neck. Lift your left shoulder off the floor by squeezing your abdominal muscles. Curl your upper torso as you move forward towards your knees. Slide your hand along your thigh until your wrist reaches your knee. Hold briefly, and lower yourself back to the ground slowly and in a controlled fashion. Keep your lower back in contact with the floor throughout this exercise, and do not pull your neck or head with the supporting hand. Do 30 seconds and repeat for 30 seconds extending your left arm and with your right hand behind your head.

Once you've completed these upper-body exercises, it's time to work on your legs.

The Second 6 Minutes

The second 6 minutes are a combination of jogging on the spot (aerobic) with resistance exercise for the legs, in the form of squats.

1. Jogging on the Spot

The aim here is not to leap and bound away, but to take relatively small steps, lifting your feet about 10 cm/4 inches off the floor.

For some people, jogging on the spot may be too intense an exercise to maintain for 6 minutes. An alternative would be to march on the spot, in which case the legs should be raised about 30 cm/12 inches off the floor. As you get fitter you may want to introduce jogging on the spot gradually into the regime until, ultimately, you're able to do this throughout.

2. Squats

Place your feet a little more than shoulder-width apart, toes pointed out slightly. Sit back until your thighs are roughly parallel with the floor (the hips should end up higher than the knees). Keep your knees over your ankles and swing your arms forward as you sit back, to keep your balance. Return to standing and repeat.

Start the second 6-minute session by running on the spot for 75 counts where you count each time your left foot hits the floor (one count equals one step with each foot). After this, immediately perform 10 squats. Repeat this sequence until 6 minutes have elapsed.

This regime is relatively brief, but it can be hard work, especially for those not used to exercise and who may be weak and unfit. Don't be too surprised, therefore, if you feel that the regime has taken a lot out of you to begin with. You can also take heart from the fact that, over time, the regime is likely to get progressively easier.

This 12-minute regime provides a great resistance workout for the upper and lower body, with some aerobic conditioning thrown in. All in the comfort of your own home or hotel room, with no special gear or equipment required save a giant rubber band or a pair of dumbbells.

How Often Should I Do This?

After being worked, muscles need time to repair. It's while they repair that muscles grow a little and get stronger, which has led to the belief that no muscle group should be exercised more than

AFFIRMATIVE ACTION

about once or twice a week. Such advice usually relates to exercises in which a single muscle group may have been worked on in the gym for perhaps an hour or more. In this time, serious damage may be caused, so no wonder it can take a week or more to recover.

Any muscle damage caused by this 12-minute session will be minor in comparison. Each muscle group is only engaged for a minute at a time, and at loads that are worthwhile but do not cause 'failure' (i.e. when you simply can't do another repetition). The recommended intensity is certainly enough to make real progress, but not enough to require days for recovery.

When you first start this programme, if you haven't done much for a while you may be a bit sore the following day and perhaps for another day or two. At the outset, let this soreness be your guide as to when to do the next session. Once your muscles have little detectable soreness, you're good to go again. In the beginning, this may mean resting for two or more days between sessions. But the fitter and stronger you get, the quicker your recovery will be. Ultimately, you should be able to do the session every day, with no soreness in between sessions.

LOW-CARB DIETS AND EXERCISE

The relatively low-carbohydrate diet advocated in *Escape the Diet Trap* may seem at odds with the carbohydrate-rich diets so often recommended for athletes. Some of you will be familiar with the concept of 'carb-loading' – the filling up on foods such as pasta and rice prior to engaging in prolonged exercise. Some say a low-carbohydrate diet risks the muscles running low on glycogen – a form of starch – which can cause energy levels and performance to crash.

There is no doubt in my mind that individuals engaging in endurance exercise might benefit from more carbohydrate in the diet compared to more sedentary people. Part of the problem, though, is that many of us eat like marathon runners but spend practically all of our time sitting on our bums.

However, even if we are not completely sedentary it doesn't necessarily make sense to load up on carbs. Let's go through some figures.

As we learned earlier, a 30-minute jog will burn about 250 calories. Let's imagine that, during the jog, 150 of the calories come from sugar and glycogen (the rest from fat). Each gram of carbohydrate contains 4 calories, so in theory to replenish the glycogen lost during exercise you are going to need to consume about 40 g of carb. That's about the same amount of carbohydrate found in a couple of apples.

In other words, for most individuals engaged in recreational, average intensity exercise that does not last more than a couple of hours, glycogen depletion is unlikely to be an issue unless carb consumption is reduced to very low levels. Even when carbohydrate levels are cut right down, remember that the body has the capacity to make it in the liver. It's estimated that the body can make about 200 g a day in this way.

Also, over time, when individuals restrict carbohydrate they become increasingly more adept at burning fat as fuel. This, sometimes referred to as 'keto-adaptation' or 'fat-adaptation', leaves individuals much less dependent on carbohydrate for energy during exercise than they might previously have been. A major review on the subject concluded that '... endurance performance can be sustained despite the virtual exclusion of carbohydrate from the human diet'.[17]

Keto-adaptation can take anything from a few days to a few weeks, so the transition to a low-carb diet is not a good idea if you are approaching a sporting event in which you want to perform to the best of your ability.

Some people find that a bit more carbohydrate is required when they engage in 'high-end' exercise that requires speed and intensity. If this is true for you, I would advise against filling up on bread, pasta and white rice. Not only are these foods generally disruptive of blood sugar levels, they also have precious little nutritional value. Generally, slower sugar-releasing and more nutritious forms of carbohydrate include fruit and vegetables, including root vegetables such as sweet potato.

AFFIRMATIVE ACTION

The Bottom Line

- Aerobic exercise is often promoted as a good way to lose weight, but studies do not support this.

- Generally speaking, exercise burns small numbers of calories.

- People who exercise more tend to eat more, too.

- Exercise may lead to people being more sedentary when they are not exercising.

- Prolonged exercise can lead to sustained rises in the hormone cortisol, which can predispose to abdominal obesity.

- Although aerobic exercise may not help weight loss, it is associated with a range of benefits for health and improved mental functioning.

- Walking has been found to have significant health benefits.

- Research shows that the benefits of exercise still exist if performed in multiple, shorter duration sessions.

- Resistance exercise can build, tone and strengthen muscle, improving body composition and the look of the body.

Chapter 22

GOING LOWER

Put into practice the advice contained in this book so far and you stand a very good chance of seeing significant shifts in your weight and wellbeing, and all without the steely determination you may have previously believed was necessary to achieve these things. However, I know from my work in practice that not all bodies respond in the same way to the strategies laid out here. A minority of people will find fat loss tough going even when there's seemingly still plenty of it to shift. Others will lose considerable amounts of weight (even quite quickly) but still hit the buffers at a weight unacceptably higher than their ideal.

This chapter offers two potential solutions to these issues – one dietary and one exercise-based. Both of them are a little more intense than the sorts of things I'd recommend for most people. However, sometimes needs must. Let's dig into these strategies, starting with a dietary strategy known as 'intermittent fasting'.

When Less Can Be More

One of the key themes of this book is that body fatness is not just about 'calories in and calories out' but is, to a large part, under *hormonal* control. A key player here is insulin, higher levels of which predispose to fatness. That is why this book advocates a relatively low-carbohydrate diet designed, among other things, to lower insulin levels.

Insulin levels can be tempered by adjusting not just what we eat, but when we eat, too. Insulin is secreted in response to eating, so it tends to be elevated during the day and relatively low while we sleep at night. In theory, extending the time each day when insulin levels are low might promote weight loss. This, in essence, is what intermittent fasting is all about.

One type of intermittent fasting is known as 'alternate day fasting'. In essence this means having food-free days alternating with days of unrestricted eating. Other forms of intermittent fasting include contracting the 'window' available for eating each day. Typically, in intermittent fasting, eating windows last from 4 to 8 hours. Don't worry if not eating for 16 hours or more seems like a bit of a stretch: there are other far less extreme ways of applying intermittent fasting that we'll be exploring later on.

The concept of intermittent fasting is relatively new, and consequently the research in the area is scant. However, what little science we have on the subject is generally positive. In one study, for instance, overweight and obese women undertook continuous or intermittent caloric restriction over a 6-month period.[1] Half the women restricted food intake to 1,500 calories a day. Those on the 'intermittent fasting' regime, on the other hand, ate 650 calories on each of two days in each week (the rest of the time they were free to eat as much as they liked). Both groups of women effectively restricted calories to the same degree (about 25 per cent of calories normally consumed).

Both groups lost weight, and also saw improvements in measures such as blood pressure and inflammation. Insulin levels fell and insulin sensitivity rose, but it did so *more* in the intermittent fasters. Improved insulin sensitivity is a good thing that should translate into improved weight loss and reduced risk of Type 2 diabetes over time. Intermittent fasting has also been linked with preservation of muscle during weight loss compared to daily caloric restriction.[2]

240

As a general rule, I believe that three meals a day is a prerequisite for healthy eating for most people, because regular eating can help keep the appetite under control and make eating healthily much easier. Yet, intermittent fasting can bring benefits, too, and if it can be done in a way that does not cause the appetite to run out of control and trigger wholly unhealthy eating, then it's certainly worth considering. While it's no panacea, my experience is that intermittent fasting often accelerates fat loss and can help individuals through a plateau.

NOT FOR EVERYONE

Intermittent fasting has merit, I think, but it's not for everyone. First of all, even if you're in a good state of health, I'd advise you not to attempt it unless you have first ensured that you are eating in a way that has effectively controlled your appetite and stabilized your blood sugar levels. Being able to delay a meal without undue hunger, having no food cravings and feeling that your energy levels are high and sustained throughout the day are all good signs in this respect. A few weeks of eating this way will also allow your body time to become better 'fat adapted' – meaning that it can subsist more readily on fat stores and is less reliant on food for energy (see below).

Those who should avoid intermittent fasting include individuals with a history of eating disorder (bulimia nervosa or anorexia nervosa) and Type 1 diabetics. Even Type 2 diabetics need to be careful here, as some adjustment of medication is likely to be required, and this should be done with support and advice from a doctor.

Others who should avoid intermittent fasting include those who are generally 'stressed' or have chronic fatigue. Stress can weaken organs known as the adrenal glands that sit on top of the kidneys and have a role to play in blood sugar balance and metabolism. In the long term, compromised adrenal function can lead to fatigue and chronic fatigue. Intermittent fasting puts further stress on the adrenal glands and is best avoided for this reason.

241

Individuals who want to improve their sporting performance should approach intermittent fasting with care, particularly if they are actively building up muscle and strength. Working with a fitness expert with experience of intermittent fasting is advised.

While our ability to go without food varies from person to person, here are two generalities that I believe hold true:

1. When someone is in the initial throes of shifting to a lower carbohydrate diet, they tend not to do well with intermittent fasting.

   The metabolic transition from a carbohydrate-rich diet to a lower carb one can take some time (usually a few days to 3 weeks), essentially because the body can need a while to get used to burning fat as its primary fuel. In such circumstances, the body can be very dependent on the maintenance of blood sugar levels and regular feeding.

2. As someone progresses with carbohydrate-controlled eating, their ability to go without food and undertake intermittent fasting improves.

   Once the body is more adept at burning fat as its primary fuel, it's less reliant on food for fuel and energy. When the body 'feeds off its fat', one's ability to go without food and not suffer undue hunger, fatigue or issues with brain function is enhanced. I've seen many individuals who, after several weeks of low-carb eating, are amazed at the length of time they can go without getting unduly hungry or experiencing symptoms such as fatigue, weakness and loss of concentration.

What to Do?

Bearing in mind that insulin levels are usually low during the night, one approach to intermittent fasting would simply be to skip breakfast or dinner. Which should you go for? My advice would be to drop the one you feel is going to be *easiest* to do without.

If you're generally hungry in the morning and find your appetite tails off at the end of the day, then I recommend skipping dinner. If you usually have little appetite in the morning, then missing breakfast would be better for you. Generally, from a social point of view I think individuals find it easier to skip breakfast. Many of us live in a culture in which breakfast is not so commonly a family or social event as dinner.

There's no reason to be rigid with intermittent fasting either. If you tend to skip breakfast, but find yourself uncharacteristically hungry one morning, my advice is to eat something. On the other hand, if you normally eat dinner but are simply not hungry one evening, this might be a good opportunity to skip it.

MY INTERMITTENT FASTING EXPERIMENT

I have personally experimented with intermittent fasting. I had been hearing good things about it so decided to try it myself. I had also been discussing intermittent fasting with someone who had lost almost 100 lbs following the low-carbohydrate and realistic exercise advice in my last book, *Waist Disposal*. She had plateaued, though, and was looking for something to get her going again. I suggested intermittent fasting, and volunteered to try it myself at the same time.

Although I have rarely skipped breakfast over the years, I am generally less hungry in the morning than in the evening. I therefore decided to go without breakfast, but resolved to do this gradually by slowly increasing the length of time in the morning before I ate anything. I generally get up quite early (6.30–7.00 a.m.), and after a week or two I found myself being able to get to 1.00 p.m. or later before I felt ready for lunch.

To be clear, I was not consciously resisting food before this time – I just wasn't hungry. I felt no decrease in energy either. If anything, my energy levels improved, particularly mental energy, focus and clarity. I also, though this may have had nothing to do with my dietary change, found myself needing less sleep.

My fellow intermittent faster found her weight loss kick-started again. I lost weight, too. Within about a month I'd lost 5–6 lbs and about an inch off my waist. I reckon my 'fighting weight' is about 140 lbs, and I normally hover around 147 lbs. In this context, losing 5–6 lbs is quite significant. My waist size shrunk noticeably, making me think that a sizeable chunk of the weight I lost was fat. At the time of writing, I usually eat only two meals a day.

Now that we've explored this dietary strategy for accelerated fat loss, let's look at a type of exercise than can help here, too.

High-Intensity Intermittent Exercise

In the last chapter (Affirmative Action) we learned that while aerobic exercise is good for a variety of things, weight loss is not one of them. In recent years, though, there has been growing interest in a form of exercise termed 'high-intensity intermittent exercise' (HIIE) that research suggests is a more efficient form of exercise for, among other things, shedding fat.

HIIE, as its name suggests, entails periods of relatively brief, intense exercise, interspersed with periods of relative rest. One typical regime uses 30-second 'sprints' on a stationary bicycle, interspersed with 'rest' periods of 3–4 minutes. Usually 4–6 of these individual cycles will be completed per session. Total session time will be about 20 minutes. During the 'sprints', individuals are usually exercising at 90–100 per cent of their maximum possible effort.

Thirty seconds of high-intensity sprinting is hard work even for highly trained individuals. Also, such intense exercise is not to be recommended for individuals who are relatively unfit or who have medical concerns that preclude hard exercise. An alternative is to reduce both the sprint and recovery times. One common protocol employs 8-second sprints, interspersed with 12-second rests for a total of 20 minutes (60 cycles).

In addition to stationary cycling, other forms of exercise that are amenable to HIIE include rowing (usually on a rowing machine) and running. I give some examples of suitable regimes at the end of this chapter.

The effects of high-intensity intermittent exercise have been comprehensively reviewed.[3] HIIE has been found to improve fitness, even in trials lasting only two weeks.

A very consistent finding was an improvement in *insulin sensitivity*. Improvements ranged from 19 to 58 per cent in the studies that measured this. Insulin sensitivity improved most, perhaps not surprisingly, in those with evidence of insulin resistance (such as Type 2 diabetics). Restoring insulin sensitivity would be expected to speed weight loss and reduce the risk of chronic illness in time.

Importantly, HIIE was also found to stimulate the metabolism of fat and fat loss, particularly in those with weight to lose.

Better than Steady State Exercise for Fat Loss?

So, in addition to other benefits, HIIE can assist speed weight loss. But how does it perform compared to 'steady state' exercise here?

In one study, women engaged in either HIIE or steady state cycling for 15 weeks. The steady state exercise involved 40 minutes of continuous exercise. In this study, HIIE came in the form of 8-second sprints interspersed with 12-second rest periods, for a total of 20 minutes. Exercise sessions were performed 3 times a week.[4]

Over the course of the study, individuals engaging in HIIE lost a total of 2.5 kg of fat. In contrast, those who engaged in steady state exercise lost *no weight at all*.

And remember, the HIIE women exercised for *half* the time.

Bigger Benefits for Health, Too

Another interesting study included in the review compared HIIE with steady state exercise in subjects diagnosed with metabolic syndrome.[5] Half the group performed 4 minutes of exercise at 90 per cent maximum capacity followed by 3 minutes of 'recovery' exercise for a total of 4 cycles. The remaining individuals exercised continually at 70 per cent maximum capacity for a similar length of time.

Fitness increased in both groups, but rose by about *twice as much* in the HIIE group compared to the steady state exercisers. Also, HIIE was significantly more effective in reversing signs of metabolic syndrome.

In another study conducted by the same group of researchers, overweight adolescents were randomized to HIIE or an approach which included exercise, dietary advice and psychological support[6] (referred to as a 'multidisciplinary' approach). After a year, the HIIE group was found, compared to the other group, to have significantly improved fitness and blood vessel function (a marker for cardiovascular disease). Plus, while waist circumference did not change significantly in the multidisciplinary group, it reduced by an average of more than 7 cm in the HIIE group.

How to Do It

Because HIIE can be very challenging, it is generally better to work up to it gradually. This helps ensure that the intensity of HIIE is not too much of a shock to the system, and reduces the risk of injury.

As with intermittent fasting, HIIE may not be for everyone. Individuals with a history of cardiovascular or lung disease or any other major illness should proceed with some caution, and only attempt HIIE once given the go-ahead by a doctor.

If you're not used to exercise, even if you are generally healthy it makes sense to build up a base level of fitness first. Brisk walking, as outlined in the previous chapter, will help, as will the

12-minute resistance-based programme also included in that chapter. It is also possible to build up a base level of fitness with light jogging, cycling (say, on a stationary bike) or on a rowing machine. After 3–4 weeks of regular exercise at reasonable intensity, you can contemplate HIIE.

High-intensity exercise is hard work, and in the beginning it is unlikely that you'll be able to sustain the 'sprints' for much more than 10 seconds. The length of the sprints can be built up over time, but for those just starting out, here are some examples of what an HIIE workout might look like.

Running:

Warm up with some gentle jogging for 2 minutes.

Sprint for 10 seconds at about 80–90 per cent maximum intensity.

Jog very gently for 30 seconds.

Repeat this cycle for a total of 6–10 sprints.

Cool down with some gentle jogging for 2 minutes.

Cycling:

On a stationary bike, warm up for 2 minutes.

Sprint at about 80–90 per cent intensity for 12–15 seconds.

Cycle slowly for 45–48 seconds (so that the sprint plus 'rest' makes up a total of one minute).

Repeat this sprint and rest for a total of 6–10 times.

Cool down with gentle cycling for 2 minutes.

Rowing:

Warm up for 2 minutes with gentle rowing.

Row hard for 10 strokes.

Row gently for 20 strokes.

Repeat this cycle 6–10 times.

Cool down with gentle rowing for 2 minutes.

Start with one of these sessions a week. As your fitness improves, you may think about doubling the frequency of sessions. As you progress, you can also make the sessions more challenging. Many different parameters can be altered here, including:

1. Putting more effort into the 'sprints' (e.g. 90–95 per cent effort).

2. Doing a greater number of sprints in total (regardless of their duration, intensity and length of rest periods).

3. Extending the time of the sprints.

4. Reducing the time of the 'rests'.

5. Extending the total session time.

Aim for gradual progression here, over weeks and months. The effort you put into this will almost certainly pay handsome returns in terms of fat loss, fitness and general health.

HIIE AND HUNGER

As we discussed in the last chapter, one of the reason aerobic exercise might not do much to accelerate fat loss is because it tends to make people hungry. While it hasn't been studied formally, anecdotally many people find that HIIE does not increase their appetite in the way more extended exercise tends to do.

The Bottom Line

- Intermittent fasting and high-intensity intermittent exercise are potentially useful tools for accelerating fat loss and helping kick-start weight loss after a plateau.

- One of the main aims of intermittent fasting is to extend the time during which insulin levels are low.

- A practical and 'doable' version of intermittent fasting is to skip breakfast or dinner.

- Individuals relatively new to low-carbohydrate eating will generally find intermittent fasting harder than those who have been eating this way for a while, and are likely to be better adapted to turning to body fat for fuel.

- High-intensity intermittent exercise (HIIE) appears to have health and weight-loss benefits beyond those that can be gained with steady state exercise.

Chapter 23

LONG GONE

One of the major goals of this book is to stop the repeated cycles of dieting and perpetual struggles with weight familiar to so many. The advice offered here is based on what science and experience tell us about how to lose weight healthily and sustainably. Because it does not entail hunger, portion control or prolonged exercise, people generally find that living this way is actually *easier* and *more enjoyable* than whatever it is they were doing that kept them at a heavier weight. That's right – you stand to achieve far better results with much *less* effort.

Yet, of course, from time to time life can get in the way of our healthy habits, and sometimes divert us from our path. Unless we lose our way for prolonged periods of time, this need not be an issue. In this chapter we're going to be looking at some of the tricks and tools that can assist you in attaining and maintaining your healthy habits as well as your improved weight and wellbeing.

Mind Control

Many people believe that establishing and maintaining healthy habits demands 'willpower' and 'discipline'. When I hear people using these words in relation to lifestyle, my heart sinks. That's because, with the *right* approach, no steely determination should be necessary. If someone is relishing what they're eating, are not unduly hungry and are finding activity invigorating but not exhausting, then why would they stop?

The fact is, believing that making healthy changes necessitates superhuman effort and self-control is misguided and just makes things harder. Having a more positive mindset works so much better.

I am a great believer that our attitudes and beliefs play a big part in our experience of life, including our health. One of the most startling examples of this is the placebo response. For example, a significant number of people given a 'painkiller' that is in fact a dummy pill (placebo) will get pain relief from it. The *expectation* of benefits does seem to have the capacity to stimulate self-healing. Could the same be true for weight and general health?

In one study, 84 hotel chambermaids were split into two groups.[1] One group was told that their work constituted good exercise, and satisfied official recommendations for maintaining health and fitness. The other group, on the other hand, was told nothing.

The women were monitored over a 4-week period, during which levels of activity remained the same in both groups. However, the group that had been told its work constituted good exercise saw improvements in several health measurements compared to the control group, including blood pressure, weight and body fat percentage. The women experienced tangible physical benefits simply because they *believed* they were doing something good for themselves.

You Better Believe It

What follows are some simple techniques designed to enhance the effects of the positive lifestyle changes you make.

See It

It's important to have a clear image in your mind of the benefits and improvements you're looking to achieve through following the advice in this book. The idea here is to move positively towards your desired outcome. This might be, for example, a smaller waist, enhanced fitness or a boost to your vitality.

The mental approach here is not the same, by the way, as not wanting to be fat, unfit and fatigued. There's an old adage: 'What you resist, persists.' So, keep your focus on positive goals, and have a clear mental picture of what these look like.

Some people who have a lot of weight to lose (say, several stone) can find they're somewhat daunted by the apparent enormity of the task they face. A useful trick can be to focus on an intermediate goal, such as getting into the next dress size or trouser size down. Once this has been achieved, a new goal can be set.

Feel It

After forming a positive image of the changes you desire, engage with this *emotionally*. Imagine what it would feel like to achieve these goals and allow yourself to get excited about it.

Be It

The final step is to act in accordance with the improved version of yourself you desire to be. Eat the health-giving foods the 'new you' eats. Engage in activities you believe the lighter, healthier version of you would take part in. Do anything and everything that is representative of the person you aspire to be.

Thinking and acting positively about your weight and health can be a powerful force for change. But there's no reason to stop there. We can also apply a similar approach to external factors, including the food we eat.

Make Friends with Food

Employing the brain as a force for good requires us to keep a positive mental attitude. Applying this principle to our diet can be especially important because many of us can build up some serious mental barriers to food. Many of us feel food has been our undoing, and this can be reinforced by messages we get about the dangers of eating certain foods. I put my hands up here: in this book I have warned you off all sorts of foods including refined sugar, starchy foods, margarine, processed fats, MSG and artificial sweeteners.

I advise against dwelling on the hazards associated with these foods, but instead focus on healthy fare. While some foods may seem to have been your downfall others, remember, can be your salvation.

In short, concentrate not on what you can't eat, but on what you *can*.

LOW-CARB – WHAT'S IN A NAME?

The type of diet advocated in *Escape the Diet Trap* certainly fits into the bracket 'low-carb'. Low-carbohydrate diets, as we've previously discussed, don't have a particularly healthy reputation in some quarters. Some people find, therefore, that there's something vaguely taboo about eating this way.

A particular conversation I had with a dietician provides a perfect example of this. We had been interviewed on a national news programme regarding the Atkins Diet (a low-carb diet) and I'd been broadly supportive of it. The dietician, however, expressed the usual scepticism.

Once we were off-air, though, she told me that a doctor at the London teaching hospital where she worked routinely recommended a low-carbohydrate diet to his diabetic patients. She hurriedly followed up this revelation with the fact that her colleague endeavoured to keep this a secret, for fear of how it would look to his peers.

One source of the negative image low-carb diets have is the propaganda that comes from groups within the food industry that rail against low-carbohydrate eating and those who support it. The fact is, the popularity of low-carbohydrate eating poses a threat to those in the business of selling high-carbohydrate foodstuffs. Therefore, I wasn't surprised (though I was a bit shocked) to receive an abusive and invective-laden email from the head of communications of the trade organization the Flour Advisory Bureau.

However, putting the politics of food to one side, I believe one reason why a low-carb diet doesn't enjoy the healthiest of food reputations has to do with its very name. The term 'low-carb' somehow suggests that such a diet is inherently imbalanced. There's more than a hint here that it *lacks* carbohydrate.

As we've learned, though, the absolute requirement for carbohydrate is none at all, which makes it virtually impossible to eat a diet that is genuinely lacking in carbohydrate. I've referred many times in this book to 'low-carb' eating, but that is not to say such a regime will leave us bereft of essential nutrients and jeopardize our health. Remember, the science shows that eating this way is not just effective for weight loss – it improves markers of health across the board.

There's No Reason to Be Rigid

Initially, I suggest quite a strict approach to the recommendations in this book. But imagine being a few weeks into your new life and significantly lighter, too, perhaps with a waistline that has shrunk by a couple of inches, and feeling fitter and healthier than you have for a long time. Does that mean you absolutely have to eschew the working sandwich lunch on Wednesday, or go without a glass or two of red wine with your dinner on Saturday night? If Friday night is 'pizza night' with the kids, should you forgo it? When celebrating a special occasion, is it not OK to indulge in a piece of cake or a delicious dessert?

There's no need to let these sorts of things derail you. In the long term, remember it's what you eat *most* of the time, not some of it, that will determine your body composition and health. The important thing here is that you do not let these incidents cloud the bigger picture. One simple mental approach that can help here is to *plan* your excursions. So, for example, if you know that Friday night is pizza night, you accept the fact that you'll be eating pizza on Friday night, but also that, once this is over, normal eating will be resumed. While writing this book, I attended a stag weekend based around drinking and golf (neither of which I do particularly well). As I was driving to the venue on a Friday, I made a mental note that come Monday morning it would be business as usual regarding my eating and drinking.

It also helps to focus not on individual meals or the odd drinking session, but on the *totality* of your diet. See whatever you eat in the context of your diet as a whole. Aim, in the long term, to ensure that at least 80 per cent of your food and drink intake comes from items in the 'consume freely' categories such as meat, fish, eggs, green vegetables, nuts, berries, water and naturally decaffeinated tea and coffee.

WHY THE ODD SPLURGE WILL NOT NECESSARILY MAKE YOU *FATTER*

Some individuals keen on keeping a track of their weight can be horrified when they find that their weight has increased by, say, a couple of pounds from one day to the next. However, it's highly unlikely this is down to the accumulation of *fat*. A pound of fat contains 3,500 calories. So, in theory, the caloric excess required to gain two pounds of fat is 7,000 calories. In the space of an evening or even a day, that would be a stretch even for someone purposefully gorging themselves on the unhealthiest foods they could find.

A much more likely cause of this weight gain has to do with accumulation of carbohydrate and water. A low-carb eating regime will generally lead to the body having lower stores of a storage fuel called glycogen (a form of starch), found mainly in the liver and muscles. If a bunch of carbs is eaten, the body can retain some additional glycogen, as well as some water (one molecule of glycogen attracts four molecules of water to go with it). A bit more salt in your supper than normal won't help matters here, either, as this can promote more fluid retention.

Basically, a bit of a splurge can register, quite quickly, as a spike in weight. On the plus side, once healthy eating is resumed, this sort of weight usually dissipates as quickly as it appeared.

Embrace Exercise

Exercise, like food, is something to which we can develop 'mental antibodies'. We may, for instance, have grown up in a school environment where exercise was used as a punishment. Or perhaps we have experience of exercise that has left us exhausted or injured. If you have put up mental barriers to exercise, the good news is that the rules have changed.

Whatever your past experiences, you can still delight in the fact that a 20–30 minute walk at lunchtime is likely to be doing you the power of good. The 12-minute regime outlined in the previous chapter need not strike fear in your heart either. In fact, you may find yourself delighting in the progress you make in terms of what you can do in those dozen minutes as the weeks go by. Even if you decide to go further, and employ some high-intensity intermittent exercise, the key thing is to see exercise as something positive, enjoyable and doable.

KEEP A DIARY

One easy exercise that can help you maintain healthy habits is to keep a diary. Each day, jot down in a notebook, on a smartphone or laptop what you've eaten and drunk over the course of that day. This simple act can help us feel more accountable for our actions, making it less likely that we're going to fall off the wagon. Another way of logging your food intake is to photograph everything you eat and drink.

At the same time, you might like to keep a brief log of the activity and exercise you have taken. It can be tremendously satisfying and motivating to look back on one's efforts here.

'Diet' Is a Four-Letter Word

For many people the word 'diet' conjures up images of restrictive, unsustainable regimes that can only take them for a few turns on the dieting merry-go-round. I strongly encourage you not to regard the nutritional recommendations here as a 'diet'. View the advice, instead, as a fundamentally healthy way of eating that mirrors the diet we evolved to eat and is in accordance with our innate physiology. It's an approach that can allow you to control your weight and enhance your health, with none of the calorie restriction, portion control or extensive exercise you may have been used to in the past. Apply the principles here, and there's no reason why the benefits you experience will not last *forever*.

However, there's no need to get ahead of ourselves. I know that many of us won't be keen to commit to change until we see the results. So, with this in mind, I suggest you resolve to give the information and advice in this book a 30-day trial. This will be long enough for you to see the benefits. How you judge the progress you've made is up to you, but what you notice may include:

• The shrinking of your waist size.

- The fit and look of your clothes, and the fact that you can wear clothes you haven't been able to get into for some time.

- The amount of weight you have lost.

- A feeling of enhanced energy and vitality.

- Improved fitness, as evidenced when being active or taking exercise.

- The satisfaction you get from seeing the distinct change in your appearance.

- Compliments from outsiders who comment on how much better you look.

- Improved self-esteem.

- More confidence in your ability to control your weight and health.

My experience is that the great majority of people who take the plunge are pleasantly surprised at the improvements they've experienced and the progress they've made within a month, and with surprising ease. From then on, continuing in this vein generally becomes a bit of a no-brainer.

As you go on, be confident that you're eating the way you were always meant to. A diet inspired by our nutritional past is what makes this way of eating future-proof. Dietary fashions come and go, but you can have confidence in the fact that your diet is not just based on science, but on common sense, too.

The Bottom Line

- A positive mental attitude can have real, discernible benefits for the body in terms of health and weight.

- Seeing and feeling the positive changes you desire, and acting in accordance with them, can accelerate your progress.

- Do not concern yourself with occasional slip-ups and indulgences: it's what you eat most of the time that's important.

- Aim to base 80 per cent of your diet on 'freely permitted' foodstuffs in the long term.

- Viewing food and exercise in a positive light can also help the process of change.

- Do not see the recommendations here as a diet, but as a tried and tested approach to weight loss and enhanced wellbeing that can be applied *forever*.

Chapter 24

ESCAPE THE DIET TRAP
IN A NUTSHELL

There's a lot of information and advice in *Escape the Diet Trap*. To make life easier for you, I've summarized the entire book here. This chapter serves as a reminder of the key points made in the book, divided up into 'dos' and 'don'ts'.

Many of the 'don'ts' serve as a testament to why conventional calorie-based approaches to weight-loss advice are so ineffective and may have failed you in the past. Be aware of these pitfalls, but don't dwell on them.

My advice is to put your energy into the 'dos' – when we focus on the things that work, we don't need to concern ourselves with things that don't.

The Don'ts:

• Don't consciously restrict calories

One consequence of this in time is a lowered metabolic rate, which can make weight loss progressively harder, even at weights far higher than is healthy. Another side effect of conscious caloric restriction is hunger, which makes change virtually unsustainable in the long term.

• Don't eat a low-fat diet

Fat is not inherently fattening and low-fat diets have been proven to be ineffective for weight loss. Low-fat diets put more emphasis on carbohydrate which drives the secretion of insulin – the hormone chiefly responsible for fat deposition in the body.

• Don't allow yourself to get too hungry

Many believe hunger is a prerequisite for weight loss. Actually, hunger makes it hard to make healthy choices and jeopardizes weight loss success.

• Don't engage in prolonged periods of aerobic exercise

Aerobic exercise such as running, cycling and rowing may promote good health, but it has limited effectiveness for weight loss. Such activities don't burn calories very quickly, and tend to make people hungrier to boot.

• Don't judge your weight according to the body mass index (BMI)

The BMI assesses the relationship between weight and height, but tells us nothing about body *composition* or the *distribution* of weight. Excess fat in and around the abdomen – abdominal obesity – is the real issue.

• Don't focus on your cholesterol level

The importance of this has been massively overstated.

• Don't buy into erroneous and misleading marketing messages

Steer clear of highly suspect processed foods that are labelled as 'diet', 'low-fat', 'zero cholesterol', 'calorie-reduced' or something similar. Such foodstuffs are marketed on faulty premises and are highly unlikely to assist you in reaching your goals.

• **Don't shop for food when hungry**

This is just asking for trouble.

• **Don't let odd slips or splurges derail you**

Put such excursions into unhealthy eating into the context of your diet as a whole. Healthy eating does not have to be 'all or nothing'.

• **Don't see the changes you make as a 'diet'**

For most people, the word 'diet' conjures up images of restriction, hunger, deprivation and unsustainability. These thoughts have no place here.

The Dos:

- Focus not on the quantity of the food you eat, but its *quality*.

- Ensure that 80 per cent or more of your diet comes from 'primal', natural, unprocessed foods such as fresh meat, fish, eggs, nuts, seeds, non-starchy vegetables and some fruit.

- Put more emphasis on fat, and less on carbohydrate, than is traditionally advised.

- Ensure that your appetite is well controlled, and that your hunger is 6 or 7 out of 10 when you eat.

- Remember, the less hungry you are, the more weight you stand to lose.

- Eat mindfully, chew thoroughly and savour food.

- Keep hydrated – keeping water by you helps a lot.

- Walk regularly, and supplement this with brief resistance exercise sessions.

- Contemplate intermittent fasting and high-intensity intermittent exercise for accelerated fat loss.

- Keep in your mind a positive image of the results you're seeking to achieve, and act in accordance with this transformation.

- See the changes you make for what they are: sustainable, enjoyable choices that stand to positively transform your wellbeing and weight.

Chapter 25

REAL-LIFE STORIES

The first two weeks of applying Dr Briffa's dietary advice were the most challenging for me, because of the sudden decrease in the intake of carbohydrate, which made up the bulk of my diet. After this, though, my body soon adjusted and it is amazing how quickly your portion size decreases

Over a 6–8 week period applying Dr Briffa's dietary advice I went from 13 stone 7 lbs to 11 stone 12 lbs. I lost weight predominantly from my upper body and mainly round my waist (which reduced by 3 inches).

It's not just the weight loss that has made this way of eating worthwhile. My energy has increased and my sleep has improved.

It was family and friends who first noticed how much better I looked – not just in terms of the weight loss, but how bright my eyes were. This is the best I have felt, physically and mentally, in the whole of my adult life.

Calum Beatt

Eating as Dr Briffa suggests has led to me being more alert, and improved my concentration and determination, too. I find myself jumping out of bed in the morning and looking forward to the day.

I've been doing a spinning class two mornings a week that has improved my fitness and helped with a knee problem. But I'll be honest and say that without the better frame of mind and motivation I probably would have just stayed in bed.

I recommend what I'm doing to others. I have a friend who decided he wanted to 'bulk up' so he started doing lots of weights in the gym. He got hungry, ate loads of carbs and got fat. I've had a chat with him and showed him my 'before and after' pics, and I think I've persuaded him that cutting the carbs and shedding fat to show off his toned muscle is the way to go.

Gareth Irvine

As an adult I had always been tall and slim, rather gangly; think Rodney from **Only Fools and Horses**. I was never unnecessarily energetic, though I enjoyed regular walking and cycling. I ate what I considered to be a reasonably well-balanced diet, drank alcohol in moderation and maintained a consistent 30–32-inch waist and 11 stone in weight. I can't say I ever actively considered my weight, diet and general wellbeing to any great extent.

This status quo continued until my mid-thirties, I think. I began driving more, and cycled and walked far less. I started to let my belt out, bought more generously fitting clothes and increasingly sat down to tie my shoelaces!

By my mid-forties I had grown a full-blown 'beer belly'/'spare tyre' and an extra chin. My weight had peaked at almost 15 stone, and I wore 36-inch-waist trousers (that's with the belly **over** the waistband!).

I was feeling rather unhappy by this time. I often felt lethargic, lacking energy and motivation though, ironically, often slept poorly. I frequently suffered with indigestion at night, became breathless on mild exertion and experienced reduced libido. Perhaps more worrying for my family and for me were the mood swings and irritability.

ESCAPE THE DIET TRAP

I recognized the need to act and to change, though I balked at diets and self-denial. I had tried the usual low-fat and low-calorie routes as well as having a number of failed gym memberships under my belt. These efforts had limited effect, often leaving me feeling hungry, tired and deprived, with little effect on my abdomen. I convinced myself that these changes were an inevitable effect of ageing and my decline into middle age.

I read an article written by Dr Briffa in one of the Sundays about weight loss. The article appeared to make sense to me and took account of a broad base of research, so I got hold of one of Dr Briffa's books. I found reassurance in the reasoning about why previous diets had not worked.

I decided to give the approach an almost wholehearted try. The cynic in me wanted to test it out, too, so I employed the diet changes detailed in the book, but made no changes to my activity or exercise and didn't completely cut out alcohol. I gave up beer and lager but continued to drink wine, mostly red.

Well, the results were impressive: with little effort and no real hardship I went from a starting point of almost 15 stone down to 12 stone 12 lbs in just five weeks. My fat loss has almost entirely been from my abdomen, though the evidence is all over me. And while it feels good to experience the loss of fat and see the numbers on the scales drop, the true benefits for me are far more profound.

I feel more energetic, I feel more comfortable 'in my skin', as it were. The feedback, comments and compliments from others have raised my self-esteem. I recognize improvements in my mood and feel more in control, less irritable and generally more positive in outlook and in my engagement with others. Oh, and libidinal concerns are well and truly resolved, too.

I don't consider myself particularly strong-willed but the results gained with this approach have encouraged me to continue. The approach is simple, intuitive and easy to follow and I in no way consider myself to be 'on a diet'.

Paul O'Rourke

REAL-LIFE STORIES

It's just over a year since we adopted Dr Briffa's dietary advice eating advice – we still can't bring ourselves to call it a diet – and we see no reason to stop now. It just isn't a diet in the usual sense of the word: there's been no deprivation, no portion reduction, no meals missed and, most significantly, no hunger.

It was a bit of a challenge in the beginning to replace the potato-shaped gap on the dinner plate, as well as our home-made breakfast loaf, but we got over it. It actually led to more creative and healthier menu planning. And at this stage it's just not an issue.

My husband Geoff dropped a stone and over 3 inches round the middle in about 6 months without any other change to his regime. I didn't need to drop any weight and made the change because it was easier to manage with the two of us eating the same meals. I didn't foresee the benefits in terms of sustained energy levels and even moods that I'd get, too. No sluggishness, no bloating, no after-dinner wipe-out for either of us.

Socially it's been much easier than you'd think. We've comfortably managed trips to Germany and the US, a holiday in Portugal and even a family Christmas, Irish-style (hold the roast spuds).

It's pretty easy once you get into the rhythm of it and the incentive to maintain it is so strong. This approach is a brilliant solution for middle-age spread – it's easy and we'd recommend it to anyone.

Ursula and Geoff Kirk

Having inclined towards portliness for most of my fifty-four years, I had pretty much accepted that it was my lot in life to be this size – not massively obese but certainly overweight, and generally lacking in energy. As a private pilot I have to have a yearly medical and at the last one my blood pressure was 138/96, and I weighed 17 stone 5 lbs. I was advised to eat less and exercise more.

Shortly after I read an article in the newspaper about effective weight loss based on Dr Briffa's work.

When I looked closely at what I ate, it was clear that while it was ostensibly 'healthy' – in that there was no junk food or sugary drinks involved – it did contain a lot of wholemeal bread, pasta and potatoes. Within two days of cutting them out I felt so much better – it was an absolute revelation. While I didn't cut carbs out altogether, they assumed much, much less significance in my diet.

I found it easy to maintain this eating regime. Three months later my weight had dropped by more than 3 stone, and my waist had shrunk from 44 to 36.5 inches. By now, my blood pressure was down to 121/84.

It is now nine months since I changed my diet and my weight is hovering around the 14 stone mark, which I only check now about once a month. I can tell just by how my clothes fit whether anything is amiss and if I feel I'm going in the wrong direction, I simply adjust the quantity of food I'm eating, or forgo that extra glass of wine.

Side benefits I have noticed are how much better I am sleeping and how refreshed I feel when I wake up, and that general 'sluggishness' that I was convinced was part of my genetic make-up is now gone. And it's so nice to receive positive comments from people who haven't seen me for a while, as to how much slimmer I am and how well I am looking.

John

At the age of thirty-eight I was the biggest I'd ever been. My friends would have described me as 'jolly' but deep down inside I was miserable and it felt like I would never be able to lose weight. I've been on countless diets since the age of eleven; some involved slimming clubs, some were drastic and some downright stupid, but I was willing to try anything so I wouldn't be the 'fat girl'. Each diet had short-term success but nothing I'd tried in the past had sustained weight loss for me. I guess you could call me a typical yo-yo dieter: lose some weight and then put it all back on again plus some more until eventually I found myself 'morbidly obese' and very unhappy with it.

I stumbled across one of Dr Briffa's books one day in a bookshop, flicked through a few pages and bought the book.

At the start I will confess that I missed bread, potatoes and pasta etc., but in a relatively short space of time these cravings subsided and I also found myself starting to feel less tired. I also used to get terrible heartburn, but as soon as I changed my eating habits, the heartburn stopped. I was also really surprised that I didn't feel hungry; every diet I had ever been on before made me feel so miserable, as though I was deprived of food.

I've never been a 'gym bunny' and have always felt very uncomfortable and out of place working out. Now, acting on Dr Briffa's advice I will get off the Tube one stop earlier on my way to work – that gives me a 15-minute walk at the start of the day and the same at the end.

I've lost a little over 8 stone, which means a total of 40 inches: 20 from my waist, 10 from my bust and 10 from my hips. I'm a lot happier, and really feel that I am in control of my diet and that my diet isn't the thing controlling me anymore.

Medically speaking, I know that this weight loss has huge benefits for me, but being a woman who cares about how she looks, the added benefit of being able to buy clothes from normal shops (not just plus size ones) and to be able to look in the mirror and actually think 'I look good' has raised my self-esteem through the roof. Lots of people comment on the weight I've lost and it's a real joy when they do. I took a photo of myself on the day I started following Dr Briffa's advice and, when I look back on it now, it affirms how far I've come and keeps me focused on the slimmer, fitter and healthier future.

NC

When my kids started calling me 'baggy belly', I knew something had to change. One Christmas, I had one of those epiphanies that I seem to get every few years as a result of catching a glance of myself in the mirror. I knew that my weight had slowly been creeping up but I never really saw how bad it was. My kids clearly did, but I had been ignoring it for a while.

I didn't want to make any half-hearted attempts to cut out chocolate, diet or go to the gym twice only never to return. I stumbled on Dr Briffa's book. I bought it and was hooked.

I embarked on my new eating regime at a weight of 101 kg and with a belly circumference of 101 cm. After a few short months I had lost 10 kg and 10 cm from my waist.

I have definitely changed my eating and drinking habits, and enjoy my new way of eating a lot as I don't feel it really inhibits me (I still have the occasional pizza or a bag of chips). I have more energy, especially in the middle of the afternoon where I used to suffer from that major drop in energy around 2.00 p.m. It was great to understand how the body metabolizes different foods, as well as having a lot of my beliefs challenged, to help me re-establish a healthy relationship with food.

On the whole, it has been a fantastic journey for me. Everyone has noticed the rapid weight loss, I feel great and have more energy. And, most importantly, the kids no longer call me 'baggy belly'.

Matt Edmundson

Learning about Dr Briffa's dietary recommendations and applying them has been a life-changing event for me. His ideas made sense to me from day one. I particularly liked the assurance that I would not have to limit my food intake provided I backed off carbohydrates and I would not have to go hungry.

My previous half-hearted attempts at dieting had always ended in failure when hunger pangs set in and overcame my willpower. This time I resolved things would be different and I set myself a target of losing at least 20 lbs and 3 inches off my waist. I achieved both targets within three months.

REAL-LIFE STORIES

In general I am now very contented with my weight, waist and general fitness. I enjoy my food and do not feel at all deprived. I was initially concerned that the large amount of fat in my diet in the form of eggs, cheese and meat might adversely affect my cholesterol levels but this has not happened. In fact, these have improved.

In addition to the weight loss, I've seen an improvement in my energy levels and wellbeing. I used to find playing 18 holes of golf would leave me noticeably tired. Now I walk 18 holes twice a week with no sensation of fatigue at all. For me there is no turning back.

Liam Ward

On adopting Dr Briffa's recommendations I was very surprised how I did not feel hungry nor did it play on my mind. What was also apparent was that I no longer felt mid-morning and mid-afternoon crashes in energy where I felt I needed something sweet to pick me up. My energy levels were much steadier and I embraced the point that you should not feel famished when you get to meal times. I tried to have a few nuts everyday at 11.00 a.m. to ensure, when lunchtime arrived, I did not overeat. I really do not miss heavy carb-filled meals and tend to feel very bloated, tired and lethargic when I do eat them now.

Eating this way means I have much more energy and none of the crashes I used to suffer. I was never fat as such, but have lost weight from my middle and am much more positive within myself and confident. My job requires a lot of presentations and meetings and feeling lighter on my feet allows this confidence to grow.

I embraced the idea that 'this is not a diet'. To me diets are pointless, and 'dieting' suggests an end date. Most diets are simply not sustainable, especially the ones my friends have tried. I saw this as a lifestyle change and embraced it fully. I now do not eat pasta, rice and bread, although I have not compromised on the odd beer. I am not a big drinker, but the Friday-night pint is still a welcome treat! I really took hold of the mindset that if you stray and eat carbs, which can be unavoidable in restaurants or at friends' dinner parties, do not be concerned or worry. Just follow it for 80 per cent or more of the time.

Mark Sumner

SCIENTIFIC REFERENCES

Chapter 1

1 Skender, M. L., et al., Comparison of 2-year weight loss trends in behavioral treatments of obesity: diet, exercise, and combination interventions, *J Am Diet Assoc*, 1996, 96: 342–6.

2 Wadden, T. A., et al., Exercise and the maintenance of weight loss: 1-year follow-up of a controlled clinical trial, *J Consult Clin Psychol*, 1998, 66: 429–33.

3 Wing, R. R., et al., Lifestyle intervention in overweight individuals with a family history of diabetes, *Diabetes Care*, 1998, 21: 350–59.

4 Brekke, H. K., et al., Long-term (1- and 2-year) effects of lifestyle intervention in type 2 diabetes relatives, *Diabetes Res Clin Pract*, 2005, 70: 225–34.

5 Wu, T., et al., Long-term effectiveness of diet-plus-exercise interventions vs diet-only interventions for weight loss: a meta-analysis, *Obesity Reviews*, 2009, 10: 313–23.

6 Shaw, K., et al., Exercise for overweight or obesity. *Cochrane Database of Systematic Reviews*, 2006, Issue 4. Art. No.: CD003817.

Chapter 2

1 Prospective Studies Collaboration. Body-mass index and cause-specific mortality in 900 000 adults: collaborative analyses of 57 prospective studies, *Lancet*, 2009, 28; 373(9669): 1083–96.
2 Pischon, T., et al., General and abdominal adiposity and risk of death in Europe, *NEJM*, 2008, 358(20): 2105–20.
3 Flegal, K. M., et al., Cause-specific excess deaths associated with underweight, overweight, and obesity, *JAMA*, 2007, 298(17): 2028–37.
4 Orpana, H. M., et al., BMI and mortality: results from a national longitudinal study of Canadian adults, *Obesity*, 2010, 18(1): 214–18.
5 Berrington de Gonzalez, A., et al., Body-mass index and mortality among 1.46 million white adults, *N Engl J Med*, 2010, 363(23): 2211–19.
6 Tamakoshi, A., et al., BMI and all-cause mortality among Japanese older adults: findings from the Japan collaborative cohort study, *Obesity* (Silver Spring), 2010, 18(2): 362–9.
7 Kvamme, J. M., et al., Body mass index and mortality in elderly men and women: the Tromso and HUNT studies, *J Epidemiol Community Health*, 2011, 14 Feb. [Epub ahead of print publication].
8 Flicker, L., et al., Body Mass Index and survival in men and women aged 70 to 75, *Journal of the American Geriatrics Society*, 2010, 58(2): 234–41.
9 Flegal, K. M., et al., Reverse causation and illness-related weight loss in observational studies of body weight and mortality, *Am J Epidemiol*, 2011, 173(1): 1–9.
10 Bouillanne, O., et al., Fat mass protects hospitalized elderly persons against morbidity and mortality, *Am J Clin Nutr*, 2009, 90(3): 505–10.

Chapter 3

1 Onat, A., et al., Measures of abdominal obesity assessed for visceral adiposity and relation to coronary risk, *Int J Obes Relat Metab Disord*, 2004, 28(8): 1018–25.
2 Feller S., et al., Body mass index, waist circumference, and risk of type 2 diabetes mellitus, *Dtsch Arztebl Int*, 2010, 107(26): 470–76.
3 Canoy, D., Distribution of body fat and risk of coronary heart disease in men and women, *Curr Opin Cardiol*, 2008, 23(6): 591–8.
4 Pischon, T., et al., General and abdominal adiposity and risk of death in Europe, *NEJM*, 2008, 358(20): 2105–20.
5 Berentzen, T. L., Changes in waist circumference and mortality in middle-aged men and women. *PLoS One*, 2010, 5(9), pt ii: e13097.
6 Whitmer, R. A., et al., Central obesity and increased risk of dementia more than three decades later, *Neurology*, 2008, 71(14): 1057–64.
7 Fisman, E. Z., and Tenenbaum, A. (eds), Impaired glucose metabolism and cerebrovascular diseases, *Cardiovascular Diabetology, Metabolic and Inflammatory Facets, Advances in Cardiology*, 2008, 45: 107–13.
8 Seneff, A., et al., Nutrition and Alzheimer's disease: the detrimental role of a high carbohydrate diet, *Eur J Int Med*, 2011, 22: 134–40.

Chapter 4

1 Keys, A., et al., *The Biology of Human Starvation* (2 vols), University of Minnesota Press, 1950.
2 Apfelbaum, M., et al., Effect of caloric restriction and excessive caloric intake on energy expenditure, *Am J Clin Nutr*, 1971, 24: 1405–9.
3 Leibel, R. L., et al., Changes in energy expenditure resulting from altered body weight, *N Engl J Med*, 1995, 332: 621–8.

4 Dulloo, A. G., et al., Adaptive reduction in basal metabolic rate in response to food deprivation in humans: a role for feedback signals from fat stores, *Am J Clin Nutr*, 1998, 68(3): 599–606.

5 Astrup, A., et al., Low resting metabolic rate in subjects predisposed to obesity: a role for thyroid status, *Am J Clin Nutr*, 1996, 63(6): 879–83.

6 Wolfe, B. E., et al., Effect of dieting on plasma leptin, soluble leptin receptor, adiponectin and resistin levels in healthy volunteers, *Clin Endocrinol (Oxford)*, 2004, 61(3): 332–8.

7 Redman, L. M., et al., Metabolic and behavioral compensations in response to caloric restriction: implications for the maintenance of weight loss, *PLoS One*, 2009, 4(2): e4377.

8 Weyer, C., et al., Energy metabolism after two years of energy restriction: the biosphere 2 experiment, *Am J Clin Nutr*, 2000, 72(4): 946–53.

9 Li Y., et al., Effects of multivitamin and mineral supplementation on adiposity, energy expenditure and lipid profiles in obese women, *Int J Obes*, 2010, 34: 1070–77.

Chapter 5

1 Tomiyama, A. J., et al., Low calorie dieting increases cortisol, *Psychosomatic Medicine*, 5 2010, 72(4): 357–64.

2 Anagnostis, P., et al., Clinical review: the pathogenetic role of cortisol in the metabolic syndrome: a hypothesis, *J Clin Endocrinol Metab*, 2009, 94(8): 2692–701.

Chapter 6

1 Bray G. A., et al., Dietary fat intake does affect obesity!, *Am J Clin Nutr*, 1998, 68: 1157–73.

2 Lissner, L., et al., Dietary fat and obesity: evidence from epidemiology, *Eur J Clin Nutr*, 1995, 49: 79–90.

3 Forouhi, N. G., et al., Dietary fat intake and subsequent weight change in adults: results from the European

ESCAPE THE DIET TRAP

Prospective Investigation into Cancer and Nutrition cohorts, *Am J Clin Nutr*, 2009, 90(6): 1632–41.

4 Pirozzo, S., et al., Advice on low-fat diets for obesity, *Cochrane Database Syst Rev.*, 2002, (2): CD003640.

5 Willett, W. C., et al., Dietary fat is not a major determinant of body fat, *Am J Med*, 2002, 113(9B): 47S–59S.

6 Klein, S., et al., Carbohydrate restriction regulates the adaptive response to fasting, *American Journal of Physiology*, 1992, 262(5): E631–E636.

7 Sabaté, J., Nut consumption and body weight, *Am J Clin Nutr*, 2003, 78(3 Suppl): 647S–650S

Chapter 7

1 Robinson, S. M., et al., Protein turnover and thermogenesis in response to high-protein and high-carbohydrate feeding in men, *Am J Clin Nutr*, 1990, 52: 72–80.

2 Karst, H., et al., Diet-induced thermogenesis in man: thermic effects of single proteins, carbohydrates and fats depending on their energy amount, *Ann Nutr Metab*, 1984, 28: 245–52.

3 Feinman, R. D., et al., Thermodynamics and metabolic advantage of weight loss diets, *Metab Syndr Relat Disord*, 2003, 1(3): 209–19.

4 Kekwick, A., et al., Calorie intake in relation to body-weight changes in the obese, *Lancet*, 1956, 271(6935): 155–61.

5 Young, C. M., et al., Effect of body composition and other parameters in obese young men of carbohydrate level of reduction diet, *Am J Clin Nutr*, 1971, 24: 290–96.

6 Rabast, U., et al., Comparative studies in obese subjects fed carbohydrate-restricted and high carbohydrate 1,000-calorie formula diets, *Nutr Metab*, 1978, 22(5): 269–77.

7 Lean, M. E., et al., Weight loss with high and low carbohydrate 1200 kcal diets in free living women, *Eur J Clin Nutr*, 1997, 51: 2 43–8.

8 Baba, N. H., et al., High protein vs high carbohydrate hypoenergetic diet for the treatment of obese hyperinsulinemic

subjects, *Int J Obes Relat Metab Disord*, 1999, 23(11): 1202–6

9 Sondike, S. B., et al., Effects of a low-carbohydrate diet on weight loss and cardiovascular risk factor in overweight adolescents, *J Pediatr*, 2003, 142(3): 253–8.
10 Layman, D. K., et al., A reduced ratio of dietary carbohydrate to protein improves body composition and blood lipid profiles during weight loss in adult women, *J Nutr*, 2003, 133(2): 411–17.
11 Samaha, F. F., et al., A low-carbohydrate as compared with a low-fat diet in severe obesity, *N Engl J Med*, 2003, 348(21): 2074–81.
12 Brehm, B. J., et al., A randomized trial comparing a very low carbohydrate diet and a calorie-restricted low fat diet on body weight and cardiovascular risk factors in healthy women, *J Clin Endocrinol Metab*, 2003, 88(4): 1617–23.
13 Volek, J., et al., Comparison of energy-restricted very low-carbohydrate and low-fat diets on weight loss and body composition in overweight men and women, *Nutr Metab (Lond)*, 2004, 1(1): 13.
14 Kennedy, A. R., et al., A high-fat, ketogenic diet induces a unique metabolic state in mice, *Am J Physiol Endocrinol Metab*, 2007, 292: E1724–E1739.

Chapter 8

1 Halton, T. L., et al., The effects of high protein diets on thermogenesis, satiety and weight loss: a critical review, *Journal of the American College of Nutrition*, 2004, 23(5): 373–85.
2 Austin, G. L., et al., Trends in carbohydrate, fat, and protein intakes and association with energy intake in normal-weight, overweight, and obese individuals: 1971–2006, *Am J Clin Nutr*, 2011, 93(4): 836–43.
3 Cecil, J. E., et al., Comparison of the effects of a high-fat and high-carbohydrate soup delivered orally and intragastrically on gastric emptying, appetite, and eating behaviour, *Physiol Behav*, 1999, 67(2): 299–306.

4 Johnstone, A. M., et al., Effects of a high-protein ketogenic diet on hunger, appetite, and weight loss in obese men feeding ad libitum, *Am J Clin Nutr*, 2008, 87: 44–55.

5 Layman, D. K., et al., A reduced ratio of dietary carbohydrate to protein improves body composition and blood lipid profiles during weight loss in adult women, *J Nutr*, 2003, Feb, 133(2): 411–17.

6 Layman, D. K., et al., Dietary protein and exercise have additive effects on body composition during weight loss in adult women, *J Nutr*, 2005, 135(8): 1903–10.

7 Nordestgaard, B. G., et al., Nonfasting triglycerides and risk of myocardial infarction, ischemic heart disease, and death in men and women, *JAMA*, 2007, 298(3): 299–308.

8 Hu, F. B., Protein, body weight, and cardiovascular health, *Am J Clin Nutr*, 2005, 82(1): 242S–247S.

9 Eisenstein, J., et al., High protein weight loss diets: are they safe and do they work? A review of the experimental and epidemiologic data, *Nutr Rev*, 2002, 60: 189–200.

10 Manninen, A. H., High-protein weight loss diets and purported adverse effects: where is the evidence?, *Sports Nutrition Review Journal*, 2004, 1(1): 45–51.

11 Poortmans, J. R., et al., Do regular high protein diets have potential health risks on kidney function in athletes?, *Int J Sport Nur Exerc Metab*, 2000, 10: 28–38.

12 Morgan, K. T., Nutritional determinants of bone health, *J Nutr Elder*, 2008, 27(1–2): 3–27.

13 Conigrave, A. D., et al., Dietary protein and bone health: roles of amino acid-sensing receptors in the control of calcium metabolism and bone homeostasis, *Ann Rev Nutr*, 2008, 28: 131–55.

Chapter 10

1 Sondike, S. B., et al., Effects of a low-carbohydrate diet on weight loss and cardiovascular risk factor in overweight adolescents, *J Pediatr*, 2003, 142(3): 253–8.

SCIENTIFIC REFERENCES

2 Brehm, B. J., et al., A randomized trial comparing a very low carbohydrate diet and a calorie-restricted low fat diet on body weight and cardiovascular risk factors in healthy women, *J Clin Endocrinol Metab*, 2003, 88(4): 1617–23.

3 Samaha, F. F., et al., A low-carbohydrate diet as compared with a low-fat diet in severe obesity, N Engl J Med, 2003, 348(21): 2074–81.

4 Foster, G. D., et al., A randomized control trial of a low carbohydrate diet for obesity, *N Engl J Med*, 2003, 348: 2082–90.

5 Stern, L., et al., The effects of a low carbohydrate diet versus conventional weight loss diets in severely obese adults: a 1-year follow-up of a randomized trial, *Ann Intern Med*, 2004, 140: 778–85.

6 Brinkworth, G. D., et al., Long term effects of a high protein, low carbohydrate diet in weight control and cardiovascular risk factors in obese, hyperinsulinemic subjects, *Int J Obes*, 2004, 28: 661–70.

7 Yancy, W. S. Jr, et al., A low carbohydrate, ketogenic diet versus a low-fat diet to treat obesity and hyperlipidemia. A randomized, controlled trial, *Ann Intern Med*, 2004, 140: 69–77

8 Dansinger, M. L., et al., Comparison of the Atkins, Ornish, WeightWatchers, and Zone Diets for weight loss and heart disease risk reduction, *JAMA*, 2005, 293: 43–53.

9 Gardner, C. D., et al., Comparison of the Atkins, Zone, Ornish, and LEARN diets for change in weight and related risk factors among overweight premenopausal women, *JAMA*, 2007, 297: 969–77.

10 Shai, I., et al., Weight loss with a low-carbohydrate, Mediterranean, or low-fat diet, *NEJM*, 2008, 359: 229–41.

11 Brinkworth, G. D., et al., Long-term effects of a very low-carbohydrate weight-loss diet compared with an isocaloric low-fat diet after 12 mo. *Am J Clin Nutr*, 2009, 90(1): 23–32.

12 Frisch, S., et al., A randomized controlled trial on the efficacy of carbohydrate-reduced or fat-reduced diets in patients

attending a telemedically guided weight loss program, *Cardiovasc Diabetol*, 2009, 18; 8: 36.

13 Wycherley, T. P., et al., Long-term effects of weight loss with a very low carbohydrate and low fat diet on vascular function in overweight and obese patients, *J Intern Med*, 2010, 267(5): 452–61.

Chapter 11

1 Boesch, C., et al., Hunting behaviour of wild chimpanzees in the Tai national park., *Am J Phys Anthropol*, 1989, 78: 547–73.

2 Goodall, J., Continuities between chimpanzee and human behaviour. In: Isaac G., and McCown, E. (eds), *Human Origins: Louis Leakey and the East African Evidence*, Menlo Park, CA: Benjamin, 1976.

3 Walker, A., and Shipman, P., *The Wisdom of the Bones: In Search of Human Origins*, New York: Alfred A. Knopf, 1996.

4 Rose, L., et al., Meat eating, hominid sociality, and home bases revisited, *Curr Anthropol*, 1996, 37: 307–38.

5 Burenhult, G., Towards homo sapiens: habilines, erectines, and neanderthals. In: Burenhult, Goran (ed.), *The First Humans: Human Origins and History to 10,000 B.C.*, New York: Harper-Collins, 1993.

6 Scarre, C. (ed.), *Smithsonian Timelines of the Ancient World: A Visual Chronology from the Origins of Life to A.D. 1500*, New York: Dorling Kindersley, 1993.

7 Ambrose, S. H., Isotopic analysis of paleodiets: methodological and interpretive considerations. In: *Investigations of Ancient Human Tissue*, Sandford, M. K. (ed.), Chemical Analyses in Anthropology, 1993.

8 Langhorne, P. A., et al., Controlled diet and climate experiments on nitrogen isotope ratios of rats. In: *Biogeochemical Approaches to Palaeodietary Analysis*, Ambrose, S. H. and Katzenburg, M. A. (eds), New York: Kluwer Academic Press, 2000

9 Ambrose, S. H., and Norr, L., Experimental evidence for the relationship of the carbon isotope ratios of whole diet and dietary protein to those of bone collagen and carbonate. In: *Prehistoric Human Bone: Archaeology at the Molecular Level*, Lambert, P., and Grupe, G. (eds), Berlin: Springer, 1993.

10 Hillman, G., Late Pleistocene changes in wild plant-foods available to hunter-gatherers of the northern Fertile Crescent: possible preludes to cereal cultivation. In: Harris, D. R. (ed.). *The Origins and Spread of Agriculture and Pastoralism in Eurasia*, London: UCL Press, 1996.

11 Bar-Yosef, 0., Earliest food producers – Prepottery Neolithic (8000–5500). In: Levy, T. E. (ed.), *The Archaeology of Society in the Holy Land*, Leicester: Leicester University Press, 1995.

12 Cordain, L., et al., Plant-animal subsistence ratios and macronutrient energy estimations in worldwide hunter-gatherer diets, *Am J Clin Nutr*, 2000, 71(3): 682–92.

13 Molleson, T.I., et al., Dietary changes and the effects of food preparation on microwear patterns in the Late Neolithic of Abu Hureyra, northern Syria, *J. Hum Evol*, 1993, 24: 455–68.

14 Angel, L. J., Health as a crucial factor in the changes from hunting to developed farming in the eastern Mediterranean. In: *Paleopathology at the Origins of Agriculture*, Cohen, M. N., and Armelagos, G. J., (eds), Orlando: Academic Press, 1984.

15 Cordain, L., Solved: the 10,000-year-old riddle of bread and milk, CAM, July 2006: 20–25.

16 National Diet and Nutrition Survey. The Office of National Statistics, 2004.

17 Kurlansky, M., *Salt: A World History*, New York: Walker and Company, 2002.

ESCAPE THE DIET TRAP

Chapter 12

1 Keys, A., Coronary heart disease in seven countries, *Circulation*, 1970, 41(supplement 1): 1–211.

2 Mente, A., et al., A systematic review of the evidence supporting a causal link between dietary factors and coronary heart disease, *Arch Intern Med*, 2009, 169(7): 659–69.

3 Siri-Tarino, P. W., et al., Meta-analysis of prospective cohort studies evaluating the association of saturated fat with cardiovascular disease, *Am J Clin Nutr*, 2010, 91(3): 535–46.

4 Skeaff, C. M., et al., Dietary fat and coronary heart disease: summary of evidence from prospective and randomised controlled trials, *Annals of Nutrition and Metabolism*, 2009, 55: 173–201.

5 Hooper, L., et al., Reduced or modified dietary fat for preventing cardiovascular disease, *Cochrane Database Syst Rev*, 6 July 2011, 7: CD002137.

6 Micha, R., et al., Red and processed meat consumption and risk of incident coronary heart disease, stroke, and diabetes mellitus: a systematic review and meta-analysis, *Circulation*, 2010; 121(21): 2271–83.

7 Hu, F. B., et al., A prospective study of egg consumption and risk of cardiovascular disease in men and women, *JAMA*, 1999, 281(15): 1387–94.

8 Quereshi, AI, et al., Regular egg consumption does not increase the risk of stroke and cardiovascular diseases, *Med Sci Monit*, 2007, 13(1): CR1–8.

9 Djousse, L., et al., Egg consumption in relation to cardiovascular disease and mortality: the Physicians' Health Study, *Am J Clin Nutr*, 2008, 87(4): 964–9.

10 Zazpe, I., et al., Egg consumption and risk of cardiovascular disease in the SUN Project, *Eur J Clin Nutr*, 2011, 65(6): 676–82.

11 Weber, P. C., Are we what we eat? Fatty acids in nutrition and in cell membranes: cell functions and disorders induced by dietary conditions. In: *Fish fats and your health*, Oslo, Norway: Svanoy Foundation, 1989: 9–11.

12 Raheja, B. S., et al., Significance of the n-6/n-3 ratio for insulin action in diabetes, *Ann NY Acad Sci*, 1993, 683: 257–8.

13 Simopoulos, A. P., The importance of the ratio of omega-6/omega-3 essential fatty acids, *Biomed Pharmacother*, 2002, 56(8): 365–79.

14 The IBD in EPIC Study Investigators. Linoleic acid, a dietary n-6 polyunsaturated fatty acid, and the aetiology of ulcerative colitis: a nested case-control study within a European prospective cohort study, *Gut*, 2009, 58: 1606–11.

15 Cordain, L., et al., Fatty acid analysis of wild ruminant tissues: evolutionary implications for reducing diet-related chronic disease. *Eur J Clin Nutr*, 2002, 56: 181–91.

16 Eaton, S. B., and Konner, M., Paleolithic nutrition: a consideration of its nature and current implications, *N Engl J Med*, 1985, 312: 283–9.

17 Simopoulos, A. P., and Cleland, L. G. (eds), *Omega-6/omega-3 Essential Fatty Acid Ratio: The Scientific Evidence*. World Rev Nutr Diet, Basel, Karger, 2003, vol. 92.

18 Noreen, E. E., et al., Effects of supplemental fish oil on resting metabolic rate, body composition, and salivary cortisol in healthy adults, *Journal of the International Society of Sports Nutrition*, 2010, 7: 31.

19 Yurko-Mauro, K., et al., Beneficial effects of docosahexaenoic acid on cognition in age-related cognitive decline, *Alzheimer's and Dementia*, 2010, 6(6): 456.

20 Pedersen, J. I., et al., Adipose tissue fatty acids and risk of myocardial infarction – A case-control study, *Eur J Clin Nutr*, 2000, 54: 618–25.

21 Ascherio, A., et al., Dietary fat and risk of coronary heart disease in men: cohort follow up study in the United States, *BMJ*, 1996, 313: 84–90.

22 Hu, F. B., et al., Dietary fat intake and the risk of coronary heart disease in women., *N Engl J Med*, 1997, 337: 1491–9.

23 Oomen, C. M., et al., Association between trans fatty acid intake and 10-year risk of coronary heart disease in the

Zutphen Elderly Study: a prospective population-based study, *Lancet*, 2001, 357: 746–51.

24 Bakker, N., et al., The Euramic Study Group: Adipose fatty acids and cancers of the breast, prostate and colon: an ecological study, *Cancer*, 1997, 72: 587–97.
25 Christiansen, E., et al., Intake of a diet high in trans monounsaturated fatty acids or saturated fatty acids. Effects on postprandial insulinemia and glycemia in obese patients with NIDDM, *Diabetes Care*, 1997, 20: 881–7.
26 Alstrup, K. K., et al., Differential effects of cis and trans fatty acids on insulin release from isolated mouse islets, Metabolism, 1999, 48: 22–9/Salméron, J., et al., Dietary fat intake and risk of type 2 diabetes in women, *Am J Clin Nutr*, 2001, 73: 1019–26.
27 Jakobsen, M. U., et al., Intake of ruminant trans fatty acids and risk of coronary heart disease, *Int J Epidemiol*, 2008, 37(1): 173–82.
28 Bendsen, N. T., et al., Consumption of industrial and ruminant trans fatty acids and risk of coronary heart disease: a systematic review and meta-analysis of cohort studies, *Eur J Clin Nutr*, 2011, 65(7): 773–83.
29 Kavanagh, K., et al., Trans fat diet induces insulin resistance in monkeys. Study presented at the Scientific Sessions of the American Diabetes Association in Washington DC, USA, 2006.
30 Gillman, M. W., et al., Margarine intake and subsequent coronary heart disease in men, *Epidemiology*, 1997, 8(2): 144–9.
31 Willett, W. C., et al., Intake of trans fatty acids and risk of coronary heart disease among women, *Lancet*, 1993, 341(8845): 581–5.

Chapter 13

1 Anderson, K.M., et al., Cholesterol and mortality. 30 years of follow-up from the Framingham study, *JAMA*, 1987, 257(16): 2176–80.

2 Scientific steering committee on behalf of the Simon Broome Register group. Risk of fatal coronary heart disease in familial hypercholesterolaemia, *BMJ*, 1991, 303: 893–6.

3 Forette, F., et al., The prognostic significance of isolated systolic hypertension in the elderly. Results of a ten year longitudinal survey, *Clinical and Experimental Hypertension. Part A, Theory and Practice*, 1982, 4: 1177–91.

4 Nissinen, A., et al., Risk factors for cardiovascular disease among 55 to 74 year-old Finnish men: a 10-year follow-up, *Annals of Medicine*, 1989, 21: 239–40.

5 Krumholz, H. M., et al., Lack of association between cholesterol and coronary heart disease mortality and morbidity and all-cause mortality in persons older than 70 years, *Journal of the American Medical Association*, 1994, 272: 1335–40.

6 Weijenberg, M. P., et al., Serum total cholesterol and systolic blood pressure as risk factors for mortality from ischemic heart disease among elderly men and women, *Journal of Clinical Epidemiology*, 1994, 47: 197–205.

7 Simons, L. A., et al., Cholesterol and other lipids predict coronary heart disease and ischaemic stroke in the elderly, but only in those below 70 years, *Atherosclerosis*, 2001, 159: 201–8.

8 Fried, L.P., et al., Risk factors for 5-year mortality in older adults: the Cardiovascular Health Study, *Journal of the American Medical Association*, 1998, 279: 585–92.

9 Chyou, P. H., et al., Serum cholesterol concentrations and all-cause mortality in older people, *Age and Ageing*, 2000, 29: 69–74.

10 Menotti, A., et al., Cardiovascular risk factors and 10-year all-cause mortality in elderly European male populations; the FINE study, *European Heart Journal*, 2001, 22: 573–9.

11 Räihä, I., et al., Effect of serum lipids, lipoproteins, and apolipoproteins on vascular and nonvascular mortality in the elderly, *Arteriosclerosis Thrombosis and Vascular Biology*, 1997, 17: 1224–32.

12 Jacobs, D., et al., Report of the conference on low blood cholesterol: mortality associations, *Circulation*, 1992, 86(3): 1046–60.

13 Alawi, A., et al., Statins, low-density lipoprotein cholesterol, and risk of cancer, *Journal of the American College of Cardiologists*, 2008, 52(14): 1141–7.

14 Yang, X., et al., Independent associations between low-density lipoprotein cholesterol and cancer among patients with type 2 diabetes mellitus, *Canadian Medical Association Journal*, 2008, 179(5): 427–37.

15 Schatzkin, A., et al., Serum cholesterol and cancer in the NHANES I epidemiologic follow-up study. National Health and Nutrition Examination Survey, *Lancet*, 1987, 2: 298–301.

16 Ulmer, H., et al., Why Eve is not Adam: prospective follow-up in 149650 women and men of cholesterol and other risk factors related to cardiovascular and all-cause mortality, *J Women's Health*, 2004, 13(1): 41–53.

17 Schatz, I. J., et al., Cholesterol and all-cause mortality in elderly people from the Honolulu Heart Program: a cohort study, *Lancet*, 2001, 358(9279): 351–5.

18 Hayward, R. A., et al., Narrative review: lack of evidence for recommended low-density lipoprotein treatment targets: a solvable problem, *Ann Int Med*, 2006, 145: 520–30.

19 Ridker, P. M., et al., JUPITER Study Group. Rosuvastatin to prevent vascular events in men and women with elevated C-reactive protein, *N Engl J Med*, 2008, 359(21): 2195–2207.

20 Cholesterol, diastolic blood pressure, and stroke: 13,000 strokes in 450,000 people in 45 prospective cohorts. Prospective studies collaboration, *Lancet*, 1995, 346(8991–8992): 1647–53.

21 Imamura, T., et al., LDL cholesterol and the development of stroke subtypes and coronary heart disease in a general Japanese population: the Hisayama study, *Stroke*, 2009, 40(2): 382–8.

22 Varbo, A., et al., Nonfasting triglycerides, cholesterol, and ischemic stroke in the general population, *Annals of Neurology*, 2011, 69(4): 628–34.

SCIENTIFIC REFERENCES

23 Kastelein, J. J., et al., ENHANCE Investigators. Simvastatin with or without ezetimibe in familial hypercholesterolemia, *N Engl J Med*, 2008, 358(14): 1431–43.

24 Studer, M., et al., Effect of different antilipidemic agents and diets on mortality: a systematic review, *Arch Intern Med*, 2005, 165(7): 725–30.

25 Weingartner, O., et al., Controversial role of plant sterol esters in the management of hypercholesterolaemia, *European Heart Journal*, 2009, 30: 404–9.

26 Danesi, F., et al., Phytosterol supplementation reduces metabolic activity and slows cell growth in cultured rat cardiomyocytes, *British Journal of Nutrition*, 2011, 106(4): 540–8.

Chapter 14

1 Scribner, K. B., et al., Long-term effects of dietary glycemic index on adiposity, energy metabolism and physical activity in mice, *Am J Physiol Endocrinol Metab*, 2008, 295(5): E1126–31.

2 Foster-Powell, K., et al., International table of glycemic index and glycemic load values: 2002, *Am J Clin Nutr*, 2002, 76(1): 5–56.

3 Bao, J., et al., Prediction of postprandial glycemia and insulinemia in lean, young, healthy adults: glycemic load compared with carbohydrate content alone, *Am J Clin Nutr*, 2011, 93(5): 984–96.

4 Westman, E., et al., Low carbohydrate nutrition and metabolism, *Am J Clin Nutr*, 2007, 86: 276–284.

5 Roberts, S. B., High-glycemic index foods, hunger, and obesity: is there a connection?, *Nutrition Review*, 2000, 58: 163–9.

6 Arumugam, V., et al., A high-glycemic meal pattern elicited increased subjective appetite sensations in overweight and obese women, *Appetite*, 2008, 50(2–3): 215–22.

7 O'Sullivan, T. A., et al., Glycaemic load is associated with insulin resistance in older Australian women, *EJCN*, 2010, 64(1): 80–87.

8 Halton, T. L., et al., Low-carbohydrate-diet score and risk of type 2 diabetes in women, *Am J Clin Nutr*, 2008, 87: 339–46.

9 Krishnan, S., et al., Glycemic index, glycemic load, and cereal fiber intake and risk of type 2 diabetes in US black women, *Arch Intern Med*, 2007, 167(21): 2304–9.

10 Barclay, A. W., et al., Glycemic index, glycemic load, and chronic disease risk – a meta-analysis of observational studies, *Am J Clin Nutr*, 2008, 87(3): 627–37.

11 Sluijs, I., et al., Carbohydrate quantity and quality and risk of type 2 diabetes in the European Prospective Investigation into Cancer and Nutrition – Netherlands (EPIC-NL) study, *Am J Clin Nutr*, 2010, 92(4): 905–11.

12 Kechagias, S., et al., Fast-food-based hyper-alimentation can induce rapid and profound elevation of serum alanine aminotranferase in healthy subjects, *Gut*, 2008, 57(5): 649–54.

13 Hollingsworth, K. G., et al., Low-carbohydrate diet induced reduction of hepatic lipid content observed with a rapid non-invasive MRI technique, *Br J Radiol*, 2006, 79(945): 712–15.

14 Samaha, F. F., et al., Low-carbohydrate diets, obesity, and metabolic risk factors for cardiovascular disease, *Curr Atheroscler Rep*, 2007, 9(6): 441–7.

15 Austin, M. A., Low-density lipoprotein subclass patterns and risk of myocardial infarction, *JAMA*, 1988, 260(13): 1917–21.

16 Faghihnia, N., et al., Changes in lipoprotein(a), oxidized phospholipids, and LDL subclasses with a low-fat high-carbohydrate diet, *J Lipid Res*, 2010, 51(11): 3324–30.

17 Volek, J. S., et al., Modification of lipoproteins by very low-carbohydrate diets, *J Nutr*, 2005, 135(6): 1339–42.

18 Brand-Miller, J., et al., The glycemic index and cardiovascular disease risk, *Curr Atheroscler Rep*, 2007, 9: 479–85.

19 Mente, A., et al., A systematic review of the evidence supporting a causal link between dietary factors and coronary heart disease, *Arch Intern Med*, 2009, 169(7): 659–69.

20 Jakobsen, M. U., et al., Intake of carbohydrates compared with intake of saturated fatty acids and risk of myocardial

infarction: importance of the glycemic index, *Am J Clin Nutr.*, 2010, 91(6): 1764–8.

21 Jakobsen, M.U., et al., Major types of dietary fat and risk of coronary heart disease: a pooled analysis of 11 cohort studies, *Am J Clin Nutr*, 2009, 89(5): 1425–32.

22 Drewnowski, A., Concept of a nutritious food: toward a nutrient density score, *Am J Clin Nutr.*, 2005, 82: 721–32.

23 Heizer, W. D., et al., The role of diet in symptoms of irritable bowel syndrome in adults: a narrative review, *J Am Diet Assoc*, 2009, 109(7):1204–14.

24 Fuchs, C. S., et al., Dietary fiber and the risk of colorectal cancer and adenoma in women, *N Engl J Med*, 1999, 340(3): 169–76.

25 Jacobs, E. T., et al., Intake of supplemental and total fiber and risk of colorectal adenoma recurrence in the wheat bran fiber trial, *Cancer Epidemiol Biomarkers Prev*, 2002, 11(9): 906–14.

26 Alberts, D. S., et al., Lack of effect of a high-fiber cereal supplement on the recurrence of colorectal adenomas. Phoenix Colon Cancer Prevention Physicians' Network, *N Engl J Med*, 2000, 342(16): 1156–62.

27 Tan, K.Y., et al., Fiber and colorectal diseases: separating fact from fiction, *World J Gastroenterol*, 2007, 13(31): 4161–7.

28 Biesiekierski, J.R., et al., Gluten causes gastrointestinal symptoms in subjects without celiac disease: a double-blind randomized placebo-controlled trial, *Am J Gastroenterol*, 2011, 106(3): 508–14.

Chapter 15

1 Lim, J. S., et al., The role of fructose in the pathogenesis of NAFLD and the metabolic syndrome, *Nat Rev Gastroenterol Hepatol*, 2010, 7(5): 251–64.

2 Le, K. A., et al., A 4-week high fructose diet alters lipid metabolism without affecting insulin sensitivity or ectopic lipids in healthy humans, *Am J Clin Nutr*, 2006, 84(6): 1374–9.

3 Shapiro, A., et al., Fructose-induced leptin resistance exacerbates weight gain in response to subsequent high-fat feeding, *Am J Physiol Regul Integr Comp Physiol*, 2008, 295(5): R1370–5.

4 Shapiro, A., et al., Prevention and reversal of diet-induced leptin resistance with a sugar-free diet despite high fat content, *Br J Nutr*, 2011, 106(3): 390–7.

5 Stanhope, K. L., et al., Consuming fructose-sweetened, not glucose-sweetened, beverages increases visceral adiposity and lipids and decreases insulin sensitivity in overweight/obese humans, *J Clin Invest*, 2009, 119: 1322–34.

6 Elliott, S. S., et al., Fructose, weight gain and the insulin resistance syndrome, *Am J Clin Nutr*, 2002, 76(5): 911–22.

7 Johnson, R. K., et al., Dietary sugars intake and cardiovascular health. A scientific statement from the American Heart Association, *Circulation*, 2009, 120(11): 1011–20

8 Vartanian, L. R., et al., Effects of soft drink consumption on nutrition and health: a systematic review and meta-analysis, *Am J Public Health*, 2007, 97: 667–75.

9 Sánchez-Lozada, L. G., et al., How safe is fructose for persons with or without diabetes?, *Am J Clin Nutr*, Nov 2008, 88(5):1 189–90.

10 Livesey, G., et al., Fructose consumption and consequences for glycation, plasmid triacylglycerol, and body weight: meta-analyses and meta-regression models of intervention studies, *Am J Clin Nutr*, 2008, 88: 1419–37.

11 Aeberli, I., et al., Low to moderate sugar-sweetened beverage consumption impairs glucose and lipid metabolism and promotes inflammation in healthy young men: a randomized controlled trial, *Am J Clin Nutr*, 2011, 94(2): 479–85.

12 Swithers, S. E., et al., A role for sweet taste: calorie predictive relations in energy regulation by rats, *Behavioral Neuroscience*, 2008, 122(1): 161–73.

Chapter 16

1 Lanou, A. J., et al., Calcium, dairy products, and bone health in children and young adults: a reevaluation of the evidence, *Pediatrics.*, 2005, 115(3): 736–43.
2 Winzenberg, T., et al., Effects of calcium supplementation on bone density in healthy children: meta-analysis of randomised controlled trials, *BMJ*, 2006, 333: 775–8.
3 Lanou, A. J., Bone health in children, *BMJ*, 2006, 333: 763–4.
4 Feskanich, D, et al., Calcium, vitamin D, milk consumption, and hip fractures: a prospective study among postmenopausal women, *Am J Clin Nutr*, 2003, 77(2): 504–11.
5 Weinsier, R. L., et al., Dairy foods and bone health: examination of the evidence, *Am J Clin Nutr*, 2000, 72: 681–9.
6 Bischoff-Ferrari, H. A., et al., Milk intake and risk of hip fracture in men and women: A meta-analysis of prospective cohort studies, *J Bone Miner*, 2011, 26(4): 833–9.
7 Bischoff-Ferrari, H. A., et al., Calcium intake and hip fracture risk in men and women: a meta-analysis of prospective cohort studies and randomized controlled trials, *Am J Clin Nutr*, 2007, 86(6): 1780–90.
8 Loones, A., Transformation of milk components during yogurt fermentation. In: Chandan, R. C. (ed.), *Yoghurt: nutritional and health properties*, McLean, VA: National Yoghurt Association, 1989: 95–114.
9 Beshkova, D. M., et al., Production of amino acids by yoghurt bacteria, *Biotechnol Prog*, 1998, 14: 963–5.
10 Östman, E. M., et al., Inconsistency between glycemic and insulinemic responses to regular and fermented milk products, *Am J Clin Nutr*, 2001, 74(1): 96–100.
11 Zemel, M. B., et al., Regulation of adiposity by dietary calcium, *FASEB Journal*, 2000, 14: 1132–8.
12 Teegarden, D., Calcium intake and reduction of fat mass, *J Nutr*, 2003, 133: 249S–251S.
13 Zemel, M.B., et al., Dairy augmentation of total and central fat loss in obese subjects, *Int J Obes (Lond)*, 2005, 29(4): 391–7.

14 Zemel, M. B., et al., Effects of calcium and dairy on body composition and weight loss in African-American adults, *Obesity Research*, 2005, 13(7): 1218–25.

Chapter 17

1 Jonsson, T., et al., A Paleolithic diet is more satiating per calorie than a Mediterranean-like diet in individuals with ischemic heart disease, *Nutr Metab (Lond)*, 2010, 30(7): 85.

2 Anton, S. D., et al., Effects of chromium picolinate on food intake and satiety, *Diabetes Technol Ther*, 2008, 10(5): 405–12.

3 Docherty, J. P., et al., A double-blind, placebo-controlled, exploratory trial of chromium picolinate in atypical depression: effect on carbohydrate craving, *J Psychiatr Pract*, 2005, 11(5): 302–14.

4 http://www.ku.dk/english/news/?content=http://www.ku.dk/english/news/dark_chokolate.htm

5 Fernandez-Tresguerres Hernández, J. A., Effect of monosodium glutamate given orally on appetite control (a new theory for the obesity epidemic), *An R Acad Nac Med (Madr)*, 2005, 122(2): 341–55.

6 Akira, N., et al., Cephalic-phase insulin release induced by taste stimulus of monosodium glutamate (umami taste), *Physiology & Behavior*, 1990, 8(6): 905–8.

7 He, K., et al., Association of monosodium glutamate intake with overweight in Chinese adults: the INTERMAP study, *Obesity*, 2008, 16(8): 1875–80.

8 He, K., et al., Consumption of monosodium glutamate in relation to incidence of overweight in Chinese adults: China Health and Nutrition Survey (CHNS), *Am J Clin Nutr*, 2011, 93(6): 1328–36.

9 Dolnikoff, M., et al., Decreased lipolysis and enhanced glycerol and glucose utilization by adipose tissue prior to development of obesity in monosodium glutamate (MSG) treated-rats, *Int J Obes Relat Metab Disord*, 2001, 25(3): 426–33.

10 Frank, G. K., et al., Sucrose activates human taste pathways differently from artificial sweetener, *Neuroimage*, 2008, 39(4): 1559–69.

11 Lavin, J. H., et al., The effect of sucrose- and aspartame-sweetened drinks on energy intake, hunger and food choice of female, moderately restrained eaters. *Int J Obesity*, 1997, 21: 37–42.

12 Rogers, P. J., et al., Separating the actions of sweetness and calories: effects of saccharin and carbohydrates on hunger and food intake in human subjects, *Physiology & Behavior*, 1989, 45: 1093–9.

13 Tordoff, M. G., et al., Oral stimulation with aspartame increases hunger, *Physiology & Behavior*, 1990, 47: 555–9.

14 Maruyama, K., et al., The joint impact on being overweight of self reported behaviours of eating quickly and eating until full: cross sectional survey, *BMJ*, 2008, 337: a2002.

15 Study presented at the Annual meeting of the North American Association for the Study of Obesity. 20–24 October 2006, Hynes Convention Center, Boston, Massachusetts, USA.

16 Zijlstra, N., et al., Effect of bite size and oral processing time of a semisolid food on satiation. *Am J Clin Nutr*, 2009, 90(2): 269–75.

Chapter 18

1 Jitomir, J., et al., Leucine for retention of lean mass on a hypocaloric diet, *J Med Food*, 2008, 11(4): 606–9.

2 Ponnampalam, E. N., et al., Effect of feeding systems on omega-3 fatty acids, conjugated linoleic acid and trans fatty acids in Australian beef cuts: potential impact on human health, *Asia Pac J Clin Nutr*, 2006, 15(1): 21–9.

3 Engel, L. S., et al., Population attributable risks of esophageal and gastric cancers, *Journal of the National Cancer Institute*, 2003, 95(18): 1404–13.

4 Sarasua, S., et al., Cured and broiled meat consumption in relation to childhood cancer: Denver, Colorado (United States), *Cancer Causes Control*, 1994, 5(2): 141–8.

5 Truswell, A. S., Meat consumption and cancer of the large bowel, Eur J Clin Nutr, 2002 (Suppl 1): 19–24.

6 Norat, T., et al., Meat consumption and colorectal cancer risk: dose-response meta-analysis of epidemiological studies, *Int J Cancer*, 2002, 98(2): 241–56.

7 Mozaffarian, D., et al., Fish intake, contaminants, and human health: evaluating the risks and the benefits, *JAMA*, 2006, 296: 1885–99.

8 Lajolo, F. M. et al., Nutritional significance of lectins and enzyme inhibitors from legumes, *J Agric Food Chem*, 2002, 50(22): 6592–8.

9 Vidal-Valverde, C., et al., Changes in the carbohydrate composition of legumes after soaking and cooking, *J Am Diet Assoc*, 1993, 93(5): 547–50.

10 Rackis, J. J., et al., The USDA trypsin inhibitor study. I. Background, objectives and procedural details, *Qualification of Plant Foods in Human Nutrition*, 1985, 35.

11 Rackis, J. J., Biological and physiological factors in soybeans, *Journal of the American Oil Chemists' Society*, 1974, 51: 161–70.

12 Divi, R. L., et al., Anti-thyroid isoflavones from the soybean, *Biochemical Pharmacology*, 1997, 54: 1087–96.

13 Gikas, P. D., et al., Phytoestrogens and the risk of breast cancer: a review of the literature, *Int J Fertil Women's Med*, 2005, 50(6): 250–58.

14 White, L., Association of high midlife tofu consumption with accelerated brain aging. Plenary session 8: cognitive function, The Third International Soy Symposium, program, November 1999, 26.

15 Chavarro, J. E., et al., Soy food and isoflavone intake in relation to semen quality parameters among men from an infertility clinic, *Hum Reprod*, 2008, 23(11): 2584–90.

16 http://www.cspinet.org/new/200208121.html

17 http://www.cspinet.org/quorn

18 Hu, F. B., et al., Frequent nut consumption and risk of coronary heart disease in women: prospective cohort study, *BMJ*, 1998, 317(7169): 1341–5.

SCIENTIFIC REFERENCES

19 Albert, C. M., et al., Nut consumption and decreased risk of sudden cardiac death in the Physicians' Health Study, *Arch Intern Med*, 2002, 162(12): 1382–7.

Chapter 19

1 Schliess, F., et al., Cell hydration and mTOR-dependent signalling, *Acta Physiol (Oxford)*, 2006, 187: 223–229.
2 Bilz, S., et al., Effects of hypoosmolality on whole-body lipolysis in man, *Metabolism*, 1999, 48: 472–6.
3 Keller, U., et al., Effects of changes in hydration on protein, glucose and lipid metabolism in man: impact on health, *Eur J Clin Nutr*, 2003, 57(2): S69–S74.
4 Armstrong, L. E., et al., Urinary indices of hydration status, *Int J Sport Nutr*, 1994, 4: 265–79.
5 Gardner, E. J., et al., Black tea – helpful or harmful? A review of the evidence, *Eur J Clin Nutr*, 2006, 61: 3–18.
6 Larsson, S. C., et al., Coffee and tea consumption and risk of stroke subtypes in male smokers, *Stroke*, 2008, 39: 1681–7.
7 Cabrera, C., et al., Beneficial effects of green tea – a review, *J Am Coll Nutr*, 2006, 25(2): 79–99.
8 Venables, M. C., et al., Green tea extract ingestion, fat oxidation, and glucose tolerance in healthy humans, *Am J Clin Nutr*, 2008, 87: 778–84.
9 Boschmann, M., et al., The effects of epigallocatechin-3-gallate on thermogenesis and fat oxidation in obese men: a pilot study, *J Am Coll Nutr*, 2007, 26(4): 389S–395S.
10 Nagao, T., et al., Ingestion of a tea rich in catechins leads to a reduction in body fat and malondialdehyde-modified LDL in men. *American Journal of Clinical Nutrition*, 2005, 81(1): 122–9.
11 Maki, K.C., et al., Green tea catechin consumption enhances exercise-induced abdominal fat loss in overweight and obese adults, *J Nutr*, 2009, 139: 264–70.
12 Golden, E. B., et al., Green tea polyphenols block the anticancer effects of bortezomib and other boronic acid-based proteasome inhibitors, *Blood*, 2009, 113(23): 5927–37.

13 Greenberg, J.A., et al., Coffee, diabetes and weight control, *Am J Clin Nutr*, 2006, 84: 682–93

14 Odegaard, A. O., et al., Coffee, tea, and incident type 2 diabetes: the Singapore Chinese Health Study, *Am J Clin Nutr*, 2008, 88(4): 979–85.

15 Van Dam, R. M., et al., Coffee consumption and risk of type 2 diabetes: a systematic review, *JAMA*, 6 July 2005, 294(1): 97–104.

16 Hino, A., et al., Habitual coffee but not green tea consumption is inversely associated with metabolic syndrome An epidemiological study in a general Japanese population, *Diabetes Res Clin Pract*, 2007, 76(3): 383–9.

17 Lopez-Garcia, E., et al., Coffee consumption and risk of stroke in women, *Circulation* 2009, 119(8): 1116–23.

18 Larsson, S. C., et al., Coffee and tea consumption and risk of stroke subtypes in male smokers, *Stroke*, 2008, 39: 1681–7.

19 Eskelinen, M. H., et al., Midlife coffee and tea drinking and the risk of late-life dementia: a population-based CAIDE study, *J Alzheimer's Dis*, 2009, 16(1): 85–91.

20 Barranco Quintana, J. L., et al., Alzheimer's disease and coffee: a quantitative review, *Neurol Res*, 2007, 29(1): 91–5.

21 Arendash, G. W., et al., Caffeine protects Alzheimer's mice against cognitive impairment and reduces brain beta-amyloid production, *Neuroscience*, 2006, 142(4): 941–52.

22 Soffritti, M., et al., First experimental demonstration of the multipotential carcinogenic effects of aspartame administered in the feed to Sprague-Dawley rats, *Environ Health Perspect*, 2006, 114(3): 379–85.

23 Van Den Eeden, S. K., et al., Aspartame ingestion and headaches: a randomized, crossover trial, *Neurology*, 1994, 44: 1787–93.

24 Lipton, R. B., et al., Aspartame as a dietary trigger of headache, *Headache*, 1989, 29(2): 90–92.

25 Walton, R. G., et al., Adverse reactions to aspartame: double-blind challenge in patients from a vulnerable population, *Biol Psychiatry*, 1993, 34(1–2): 13–17.

26 http://www.dorway.com/peerrev.html

27 Lukasiewicz, E., et al., Alcohol intake in relation to body mass index and waist-to-hip ratio: the importance of type of alcoholic beverage, *Public Health Nutr*, 2005, 8(3): 315–20.
28 Dallongeville, J., et al., Influence of alcohol consumption and various beverages on waist girth and waist-to-hip ratio in a sample of French men and women, *Int J Obes Relat Metab Disord*, 1998, 22(12): 1178–83.
29 Wannamethee, S. G., et al., Alcohol and adiposity: effects of quantity and type of drink and time relation with meals, *Int J Obes (Lond)*, 2005, 29(12): 1436–44.
30 White, I.R., et al., Alcohol consumption and mortality: modelling risks for men and women at different ages, *BMJ*, 2002, 325: 191.
31 McCann, S. E., et al., Alcoholic beverage preference and characteristics of drinkers and nondrinkers in western New York (United States), *Nutr Metab Cardiovasc Dis*, 2003, 13(1): 2–11.
32 Tjonneland, A. M., et al., The connection between food and alcohol intake habits among 48, 763 Danish men and women. A cross-sectional study in the project 'Food, cancer and health', *Ugeskr Laeger*, 1999, 161(50): 6923–7.
33 Barefoot, J. C., et al., Alcohol beverage preference, diet and health habits in the UNC Alumni Heart Study, *Am J Clin Nutr*, 2002, 76(2): 466–72.

Chapter 21

1 Melanson, E. L., et al., Exercise improves fat metabolism in muscle but does not increase 24-h fat oxidation, *Exerc Sport Sci Rev*, 2009, 37(2): 93–101.
2 Finlayson, G., et al., Acute compensatory eating following exercise is associated with implicit hedonic wanting for food, *Physiology & Behavior*, 2009, 97(1): 62–7.
3 Goran, M. I., et al., Endurance training does not enhance total energy expenditure in healthy elderly persons, *Am J Physiol*, 1992, 263: 950–57.

4 Meijer, E. P., et al., Effect of exercise training on total daily physical activity in elderly humans, *Eur J Appl Physiol Occup Physiol*, 1999, 80: 16–21.

5 Morio, B., et al., Effects of 14 weeks of progressive endurance training on energy expenditure in elderly people, *Br J Nutr*, 1998, 80: 511–19.

6 Manthou, E., et al., Behavioral compensatory adjustments to exercise training in overweight women, *Medicine & Science in Sports & Exercise*, 2010, 42(6): 1121–8.

7 Metcalf, B. S., et al., Fatness leads to inactivity, but inactivity does not lead to fatness: a longitudinal study in children (EarlyBird 45), *Arch Dis Chil*, 2011, 96(10): 942–7.

8 Catenacci, V.A., et al., The role of physical activity in producing and maintaining weight loss, *Nat Clin Pract Endocrinol Metab*, 2007, 3(7): 518–29.

9 Van der Heijden, G. J., et al., A 12-week aerobic exercise program reduces hepatic fat accumulation and insulin resistance in obese, hispanic adolescents, *Obesity* (Silver Spring), 2010, 18(2): 384–90.

10 Voss, M. W., et al., Plasticity of brain networks in a randomized intervention trial of exercise training in older adults. Frontier in Aging Neuroscience, 2010, 26; 2.

11 Miyashita, M., et al., Accumulating short bouts of brisk walking reduces postprandial plasma triacylglycerol concentrations and resting blood pressure in healthy young men, *Am J Clin Nutr*, 2008, 88(5): 1225–31.

12 Schmidt, W. D., et al., Effects of long versus short bout exercise on fitness and weight loss in overweight females, *J Am Coll Nutr*, 2001, 20(5): 494–501.

13 Bravata, D. M., et al., Using pedometers to increase physical activity and improve health: a systematic review, *JAMA*, 2007, 298(19): 2296–304.

14 Wycherley, T. P., et al., A high-protein diet with resistance exercise training improves weight loss and body composition in overweight and obese patients with type 2 diabetes, *Diabetes Care*, 2010, 33(5): 969–76.

15 Geliebter, A., et al., Effects of strength or aerobic training on body composition, resting metabolic rate, and peak oxygen consumption in obese dieting subjects, *Am J Clin Nutr*, 1997, 66(3): 557–63.
16 Stiegler, P., et al., The role of diet and exercise for the maintenance of fat-free mass and resting metabolic rate during weight loss, *Sports Med*, 2006, 36(3): 239–62.
17 Phinney, S. D., Ketogenic diets and physical performance, *Nutr Metab (Lond)*, 2004; 1.

Chapter 22

1 Harvie, M. N., et al., The effects of intermittent or continuous energy restriction on weight loss and metabolic disease risk markers: a randomized trial in young overweight women, *Int J Obes (Lond)*, 5 Oct, 2011, 118(5): 111–25.
2 Varady, K. A., Intermittent versus daily calorie restriction: which diet regimen is more effective for weight loss? *Obesity Reviews*. Article first published online: 16 March 2011.
3 Boutcher, S. H., et al., High-intensity intermittent exercise and fat loss, *Journal of Obesity*, 2011, 12(7): e593–601.
4 Trapp, E. G., et al., The effects of high-intensity intermittent exercise training on fat loss and fasting insulin levels of young women, *Int J Obes (Lond)*, 2008, 32(4): 684–91.
5 Tjønna, A. E., et al., Aerobic interval training versus continuous moderate exercise as a treatment for the metabolic syndrome: a pilot study, *Circulation*, 2008, 118(4): 346–54.
6 Tjønna, A. E., et al., Aerobic interval training reduces cardiovascular risk factors more than a multitreatment approach in overweight adolescents, *Clinical Science*, 2009 116(4): 317–26.

Chapter 23

1 Crum, A. J., et al., Mind-set matters: exercise and the placebo effect, *Psychol Sci*, 2007, 18(2): 165–71.

ABOUT THE AUTHOR

Dr John Briffa BSc (Hons) MB BS

Dr John Briffa is a medical doctor, author and speaker. He is a prize-winning graduate of University College London School of Medicine and a leading authority on diet, weight management and natural health.

A recipient of the Health Journalist of the Year award in the UK, Dr Briffa is a former columnist for the *Daily Mail* and the *Observer*, and has contributed to a wide range of newspaper and magazine titles including *The Times, The Telegraph, Men's Health, Psychologies, Options, Zest* and *Reader's Digest. Escape the Diet Trap* is Dr Briffa's eighth book.

Dr Briffa is a specialist in wellbeing and effectiveness in the workplace. He regularly delivers talks and courses on how individuals can use simple lifestyle adjustments to optimise their energy, effectiveness and personal sustainability. Clients include Deloitte, PricewaterhouseCoopers, Norton Rose, IBM, Bank of England, Morgan Stanley, Baker and Mackenzie, Bovis Lend Lease, Danone, Clifford Chance, Eversheds, GE Money, Skandia, SSL International and Reuters.

For more details about Dr John Briffa and his work see www.drbriffa.com

Contact details:

Dr John Briffa can be contacted at:

Woolaston House
17–19 View Road
Highgate
London
N6 4DJ
UK
Tel: +44 (0) 208 341 3422
Fax: +44 (0) 208 340 1376
Email: john@drbriffa.com

Dr John Briffa's website – www.drbriffa.com – includes more than 1,000 blog posts and podcasts.

RESOURCES

While I'd like to take the credit for all of the ideas expressed in this book, in reality they are a fusion of concepts that have come from a wide variety of sources. At least some of the concepts here have come from reading the work of dedicated writers and bloggers. What follows is a list, in no particular order, of the blogs I read and follow most regularly. I can't claim that I agree with every idea they express, but I have found all of them a valuable source of information and inspiration.

Dr William Davis
Bill is a practising cardiologist in the US. While he has a specific interest in heart health, his blog covers an eclectic range of health topics.

www.trackyourplaque.com/blog

Mark Sissons

Mark is an ex-marathon runner and a proponent of 'primal' living, particularly with regard to diet and exercise. His website is a great all-round resource for those looking to take control of their health.

www.marksdailyapple.com

Petro (Peter) Dobromylskyj

Peter is a practising vet, and writes a very thoughtful, considered blog with a strong nutrition bent. It was Peter who opened my eyes to the idea that effective fat loss can quell appetite and help individuals lose weight without hunger.

www.high-fat-nutrition.blogspot.com

Robb Wolf

Robb is the author of *The Paleo Solution* and an advocate of living in accordance with our ancient ancestry.

www.robbwolf.com

Dr Stephan Guyenet

Stephan researches the neurobiology of body fat regulation and obesity. His blog is well-researched and a good read. Reading Stephan's work impressed on me the importance of the hormone leptin in body weight control.

www.wholehealthsource.blogspot.com

Jimmy Moore

Jimmy is a big low-carb advocate, and his blogs and podcasts have introduced me to some great information and the work of other bloggers and researchers.

www.livinlavidalowcarb.com

Dr Emily Deans

Emily is a psychiatrist searching for 'evolutionary solutions to the general and mental health problems of the 21st century'.

www.evolutionarypsychiatry.blogspot.com

Angelo Coppola

Angelo is responsible for the podcast-based blog known as *Latest in Paleo*. Here, he presents regular, interesting and entertaining information on diet and exercise. Always a really good listen.

www.latestinpaleo.com

Tom Naughton

Tom is a comedian and creator of the movie *Fat Head*. I find his blog educational and entertaining in roughly equal measure.

www.fathead-movie.com

Professor Richard Feinman

Richard is Professor of Biochemistry at Downstate Medical Center (SUNY) in New York. His scientific publications have been particularly valuable to me in my understanding of the potential for certain diets to have metabolic advantage (see Chapter 7).

www.rdfeinman.wordpress.com

Gary Taubes

Gary is an award-winning science writer and author of the best-selling books *Good Calories, Bad Calories* (titled *The Diet Delusion* in the UK) and *Why We Get Fat*.

www.garytaubes.com

Denise Minger
Denise originally started her blog to 'combat some of the health myths floating around the vegan and raw-food diet spheres'. She, I think, specialises in thorough but entertaining analysis of nutritional concepts and the revealing of untruths.

www.rawfoodsos.com

Chris Masterjohn
Chris is a debunker of myth and misinformation in the area of nutrition. He takes a research-based and objective eye to the topic.

www.cholesterol-and-health.com

Richard Nikoley
Richard writes a good and irreverent blog covering nutrition and exercise information.

www.freetheanimal.com

Dr Mike Eades
Mike is co-author (with his wife) of the best-selling book *Protein Power*. His blog is a great resource for information and analysis of the evidence on all aspects of diet and nutrition.

www.proteinpower.com

Todd Becker
Todd has an engineering background and writes a thought-provoking blog about a wide range of health-related matters including nutrition.

www.gettingstronger.org

ACKNOWLEDGEMENTS

Robert Kirby, my fantastic agent, for being a pleasure to work with and a true friend.

Dr Peter Robbins, Nicky Chapman, Glenn Whitney and Sara Neill, all of whom made invaluable and massively appreciated comments on drafts of the book. The final result is a lot better for their input.

Richard Collins, my editor, for giving the book some much-needed spit and polish.

Chris Williams, Chris Swain, Charlie Cannon and Matt Blakely, for their help and advice regarding the exercise routine in chapter 21.

My parents – Dr Joseph Briffa and Dr Dorothy Burgess – for their enduring love, support and encouragement.

And Sandra, for her love, kindness, support and understanding.

Also, I'd like to thank the researchers, writers and bloggers who have contributed to the field and my knowledge and understanding. Please see the resources section for a list of the writers and bloggers that I read regularly and recommend.

INDEX

ESCAPE THE DIET TRAP

INDEX

ESCAPE THE DIET TRAP

314